Infection and Immunity, second edition

John H.L. Playfair

Emeritus Professor of Immunology,
University College London Medical School

Gregory J. Bancroft

Reader in Immunology,
Department of Infectious and Tropical Diseases,
London School of Hygiene and Tropical Medicine

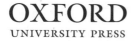

OXFORD

UNIVERSITY PRESS

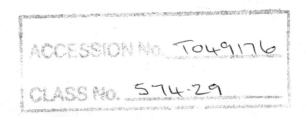

OXFORD
UNIVERSITY PRESS

Great Clarendon Street, Oxford OX2 6DP
Oxford University Press is a department of the University of Oxford.
It furthers the University's objective of excellence in research, scholarship,
and education by publishing worldwide in

Oxford New York

Auckland Cape Town Dar es Salaam Hong Kong Karachi
Kuala Lumpur Madrid Melbourne Mexico City Nairobi
New Delhi Shanghai Taipei Toronto

With offices in

Argentina Austria Brazil Chile Czech Republic France Greece
Guatemala Hungary Italy Japan South Korea Poland Portugal
Singapore Switzerland Thailand Turkey Ukraine Vietnam

Oxford is a registered trade mark of Oxford University Press
in the UK and in certain other countries

Published in the United States
by Oxford University Press Inc., New York

First published 2004
Reprinted 2005

A catalogue record for this book is available from the British Library

Library of Congress Cataloging in Publication Data
Data available

ISBN - 13: 978-0-19-926495-7
ISBN - 10: 0-19-926495-3
2
Typeset by SNP Best-set Typesetter Ltd., Hong Kong
Printed in Great Britain by
Antony Rowe Ltd., Chippenham, Wiltshire

Preface to the first edition

Infectious disease is something that affects and surely interests everyone, but for a clear picture of what actually happens during an infection, it is usually necessary to consult one or more large textbooks, since the subject falls across the conventional disciplines of microbiology, immunology, pathology, pharmacology, epidemiology, and medicine.

In this book I have tried to summarize the essentials in a way that can be understood by any student or potential student of science or medicine, including (I hope) the sixth-former and the interested layman. The content of the book corresponds roughly to the second-year BSc course 'Immunity to Infection' run at University College, London, and presupposes no previous knowledge of either microbiology or immunology. The style has been kept as close as possible to actual lectures and tutorials, including an element of self-testing and a guide to the books that can, if desired, be used for delving deeper into the subject.

Both style and content have largely been shaped by the students who have taken the course and made their comments, and I have to thank them for such virtues as it may have. Any errors are, of course, my own, and I would be grateful to be told about them. I also want to thank my colleagues at UCL for many useful suggestions, and my editors at Oxford University Press for their faith in the venture.

London   J.H.L.P.
November 1994

Preface to the second edition

The first edition of this book was intended as a compact text to accompany science courses (e.g. 2nd year BSc, MSc) for any student who needed to know something about immunity and its basis in infectious disease. There was not, and still is not, any other text of comparable length that covers the subject at the same level.

Eight years later, the text obviously needed radical updating—in particular the areas of innate immune mechanisms, microbial genomics, and AIDS, which have undergone a veritable revolution. We have taken the opportunity to extend the coverage of these whole topics, and also to provide much more detail in the opening microbiology section (enlarged from one chapter to six), which some teachers felt was too brief to balance the mainly immunological section: the section on prion diseases has obviously been expanded beyond all recognition. We have also increased the coverage of disease control, including epidemiology, and provided three new appendices listing important pathogens, cytokines, and CD molecules, while the previous appendix on immunity to ten selected infections has been upgraded to five substantial chapters, in which the preceding material on infectious organisms and the immune system is brought together into a summary of the present situation with respect to all the common and important human infections. As far as possible we have retained the concept that one chapter corresponds roughly to one 50-minute lecture, so that the book can easily be adapted to a typical unit or half-unit course. To facilitate this, all figures and tables are available from the accompanying website.

As a result the book is considerably longer, but we should stress that its aims have not changed. It is not a textbook of microbiology or immunology, but an integration of the two disciplines into a readable, accurate, and up-to-date account of how infectious disease is caused and controlled, intelligible to any science student (or ex-student).

JHL Playfair
GJ Bancroft

Acknowledgements

We are grateful to the following colleagues for useful comments and contributions to this new edition: Quentin Bickle, Dorothy Crawford, Simon Croft, Andy Hall, Catherine Hawrylowicz, Paul Kaye, John Raynes, Silke Schelenz, Debbie Smith, Richard Titball, Brendan Wren.

The role of the infinitely small is infinitely large.

Louis Pasteur

Contents

Part 3   The host–pathogen balance

Abbreviations

AFB	acid fast bacilli
ADA	adenosine deaminase
ADCC	antibody-dependent cellular cytotoxicity
AIDS	acquired immune deficiency syndrome
APC	antigen-presenting cells
ARC	AIDS-related complex
ARDS	adult respiratory distress syndrome
ATP	adenosine triphosphate
BALT	bronchi-associated lymphoid tissue
BCG	bacille Calmette-Guérin
BCR	B cell receptor
BSE	bovine spongiform encephalopathy
C	constant (gene); also complement
cAMP	cyclic adenosine monophosphate
CD	cluster of differentiation
CDR	complementarity-determining regions
CGD	chronic granulomatous disease
CJD	Creutzfeldt–Jakob disease
CLL	chronic lymphoid leukaemia
CMC	chronic mucocutaneous candidiasis
CMV	cytomegalovirus
CNS	central nervous system
CRP	C-reactive protein
CTL	cytotoxic T lymphocyte
D	diversity (gene)
dATP	deoxyadenosine triphosphate
DC	dendritic cells
dGTP	deoxyguanosine triphosphate

DIC	disseminated intravascular coagulation
DTH	delayed-type hypersensitivity
EBV	Epstein–Barr virus
EHEC	enterohaemorrhagic *Escherichia coli*
EIEC	enteroinvasive *Escherichia coli*
ELISA	enzyme-linked immunosorbent assay
EPEC	enteropathogenic *Escherichia coli*
ER	endoplasmic reticulum
ETEC	enterotoxic *Escherichia coli*
Fab	antigen-binding fragment (immunoglobulin)
Fc	crystallizable fragment (immunoglobulin)
GALT	gut-associated lymphoid tissue
GM-CSF	granulocyte and macrophage colony-stimulating factor
gp	glycoprotein
GPI	glycosyl-phosphatidylinositol
GVH	graft-versus-host (disease)
HAART	highly active anti-retroviral therapy
HEV	high endothelial venule
HHV	human herpes virus
HIV	human immunodeficiency virus
HLA	human leucocyte antigen
HSV	herpes simplex virus (HSV1, HSV2)
HTLV	human T cell lymphotropic virus (HTLV-1, HTLV-2)
ICAM	intercellular adhesion molecule
IFN	interferon
IL	interleukin
ISCOMs	immunostimulating complexes
J	joining (gene)
KIR	killer cell Ig-like receptors
LFA	lymphocyte function antigen
LGL	large granular lymphocytes
LPAM	lamina propria-associated molecule
LPS	lipopolysaccharide
LT	leukotrienes
LTR	long terminal repeat
mAbs	monoclonal antibodies

MALT	mucosa-associated lymphoid tissue
MASP	MBP-associated serine protease
MBL	mannose-binding lectin
MBP	major basic protein
MHC	major histocompatibility complex
MPO	myeloperoxidase
MRSA	methicillin-resistant *Staphylococcus aureus*
NAD	nicotinamide–adenine dinucleotide
NHL	non-Hodgkin's lymphoma
NK	natural killer (cell)
PAMP	pathogen-associated molecular patterns
PAS	*p*-aminosalicylic acid
PG	prostaglandins
PHA	phytohaemagglutinin
PMN	polymorphonuclear leucocyte
PNP	purine nucleoside phosphorylase
PPD	purified protein derivative
PrPs	prion proteins
ROI	reactive oxygen intermediates
RSV	respiratory syncytial virus
SAP	serum amyloid P
SARS	severe acute respiratory syndrome
SCF	stem cell factor
SCID	severe combined immunodeficiency
SIV	simian immunodeficiency virus
SLP1	secretory leukoproteinase inhibitor
SP	surfactant protein (SP-A, SP-D)
TAP	transporters associated with antigen processing
TB	tuberculosis
TCR	T cell receptor
T_H	T helper cell (T_H1, T_H2)
Ti	T-independent (antigen)
TD	T-dependent
TNF	tumour-necrosis factor
TSE	transmissible spongiform encephalopathies
TSH	thyroid-stimulating hormone

V	variable (gene)
VCAM	vascular cell adhesion molecule
vCJD	new variant CJD
VLA	very late activation (antigen)
VSG	variant-specific glycoprotein
VZV	varicella zoster virus
ZN	Ziehl–Neelsen (stain)

Part 1

The infectious organisms

1 Introduction: parasites, pathogens, and immunity

For thousands of years it was known that many of our most serious diseases could be caught from another individual but only with the invention of the microscope in the seventeenth century and the work of Pasteur and Koch 200 years later was it realized that these *infectious* diseases were caused by the transfer from person to person of infectious *organisms*, invisible parasites living in the body of a much larger host. However, it was also soon realized that the presence of such parasites by no means always caused disease (in this book those that do will generally be referred to as *pathogens*). So before embarking on the study of infectious organisms (microbiology) and the means by which the host can try to control them (immunology) it is worth briefly considering parasitism itself. Why are there parasites? What do they want? Is it better to be a parasite or not? Why do some parasites cause disease while others are harmless?

Our planet is a crowded place, and animals cannot help coming in contact with members of their own and other species. From the very beginning of animal evolution, such contacts have posed important questions, mostly of the yes-or-no type such as, 'is it food?' or, in the case of colonial organisms such as corals and sponges, 'to fuse or not to fuse?' (Fig. 1.1). As will be seen later, decisions of this kind, turning on the key distinction between *self* and *not-self*, are still central to immunology, even in the most advanced animals.

With larger animals, the options for interaction are quite numerous. Another species may be treated as prey and taken in as dead meat, or if small enough it may succeed in getting in alive and surviving as a resident. Here the relationship may be convenient to the host (*mutualism*), of neutral value (*commensalism*), or definitely inconvenient (*parasitism*) (Fig. 1.2). The study of infectious disease concerns, for the most part, the last situation. Note that the traditional use of the term 'parasite' to refer only to tropical protozoa and worms is fairly illogical and unhelpful; a virus is no less a parasite (indeed more so) than a roundworm, and as mentioned above, in this book the term *pathogen* will be used for all those microorganisms that get into larger animals and do harm of some kind. It is interesting that Pasteur's definition of a virus was 'a small obligate parasite requiring energy and information from a host organism'.

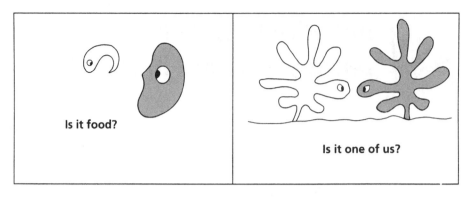

Fig. 1.1 Protozoa considering items of food, or colonies of coral in a position to undergo fusion, make recognition decisions quite similar to those that are the responsibility of the immune system in higher animals.

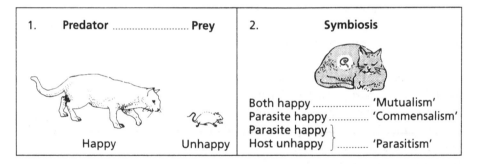

Fig. 1.2 Various two-partner relationships. The study of infectious disease is chiefly about the relationship between host and parasite (pathogen).

Pathogens

You do not need to be an expert microbiologist to understand infection, but you do need to know certain facts about the five classes of pathogens that cause infectious disease—the *viruses*, *bacteria*, *fungi*, *protozoa*, and *helminths* (worms), together with those strange bits of infectious protein, the *prions*. A sixth class, the insects inhabiting the skin (ectoparasites), will not be considered here since they remain outside the body although they can engage the attention of the immune system. However, some insects and other animals will feature in later sections as *vectors* or alternative hosts for some pathogens.

In fact, the terms 'microorganism' and 'microbe' are slightly ambiguous, implying something you need a microscope to see, which does not apply to most of the parasitic worms. It is interesting to compare the sizes of the major parasites of interest to man, which range over 9 orders of magnitude (Fig. 1.3). Note that the largest ones are much closer in size to man than they are to the smallest ones,

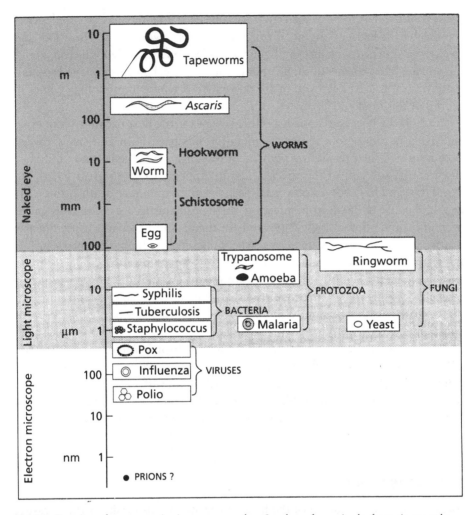

Fig. 1.3 Parasites of man range in size over more than 9 orders of magnitude, from viruses only visible in the electron microscope to worms easily visible to the naked eye. One important distinction is between those too big to be taken in by phagocytes (worms and the largest fungi) and those small enough to be disposed of in this way (all the rest). Another is between those incapable of independent existence (e.g. viruses) and the rest.

so it is not surprising that they too have their parasites—right down to the bacteria, which can be infected with special viruses known as bacteriophages.

Some of the advantages of being a parasite are obvious. As a parasite you are protected from the hostile conditions of the outside world (heat, cold, injury, etc.); you are provided with many of your nutritional needs and synthetic pathways; you can travel over relatively great distances without exertion (many tropical parasites use insects for this purpose); you can therefore devote much of your efforts to reproduction. On the down side, you are obliged to go where your host goes; your diet has to be chosen from what he eats; you may have to use ingenuity to enter the host, to migrate through his tissues to your chosen location, and to exit again in order to spread; if your host dies you are likely to die too; above all, you are likely to encounter formidable defence mechanisms designed to eliminate you or at least keep you in check—which is where immunology comes in (Part 2 of this book).

Death of the host is of course a critical event for the host organism too, especially if it occurs before the next generation has been born and safely raised, because it will then result in a permanent loss of parental genes and ultimately threaten the survival of the species. Nature appears to go to great lengths to avoid this, and has evolved powerful mechanisms to minimize death at this early age. In the case of death from infection, these mechanisms are collectively called *immunity*, and immunology is the study of them. Another major cause of early deaths, injury, is similarly prevented where possible by the *healing* process. It is interesting that the mechanisms for preventing the main causes of death in old age, degenerative disease and cancer, are much less well developed—which is perfectly logical when it is considered that, with the possible exception of humans, elderly members of most animal species are usually a burden, in terms of consumption versus productivity.

The five classes of organism mentioned above display a huge range of variation, between and within classes. Some of the characteristics of an organism that can influence the pattern of infection it causes and the effectiveness or otherwise of immunity are listed in Table 1.1. Those that facilitate infection are often lumped together as *virulence factors*, and we shall return to these in Chapter 8.

Infectious disease

As mentioned earlier, death of the host constitutes a grave risk for the parasite, but what about *disease*? One could argue that the ideal parasite would not cause its host to die or develop disease, and certainly there are examples of this idyllic

Table 1.1 Both infection and immunity are influenced by particular features of the pathogen concerned

Affecting infection	Affecting immunity
Means of entry and spread	Habitat (intracellular or extracellular)
Rate of multiplication (if any)	Susceptibility to immune mechanisms
Ability to damage tissue	Ability to escape immune mechanisms
Ease of transmission to other hosts	Ability to damage the immune system
Existence of animal reservoir	
Drug therapy (if any)	Suitability for vaccination

coexistence, including the millions of bacteria that reside harmlessly, and even beneficially, in our intestinal tract. But the parasites we are most interested in are precisely those that *do* cause disease, the pathogens, which unfortunately are very numerous and widespread and a major cause of death, particularly in tropical countries (see Table 1.2). Why have they not achieved the 'ideal' state? This is a very deep question to which there is no easy answer. It used to be assumed that all parasite–host combinations would, given time, evolve towards the ideal state, or at least to a state where they did not kill the host. According to this theory, parasites that frequently did kill their hosts were simply not yet properly 'adapted'. Again, examples can be found, such as the fact that the often fatal human malaria parasite, *Plasmodium falciparum*, appears to have got into man (probably from birds) more recently than the other three milder species of malaria, which reached us via other primates. A similar argument is based on 'zoonotic' infections, such as plague, Lassa fever, and the immunodeficiency viruses, that are still mainly restricted to animals and so have not had to adapt to man. When they do infect man they are very often fatal; in one of these, human immunodeficiency virus (HIV), we have had the dubious privilege of actually being able to follow the genetic evolution of the virus as it spread from primates to man. However, experts in this field, modelling millions of years of host–parasite evolution on their computers, no longer accept the old generalization. Each parasite–host combination has to be looked at separately; sometimes

Table 1.2 Infectious diseases are now a relatively minor cause of death in developed countries, but still extremely important elsewhere

Cause of death	Deaths per year (approximately)	
	Industrialized countries	Developing countries
Circulatory disease	5 900 000	6 500 000
Cancer	2 300 000	2 500 000
Infectious disease	500 000	16 500 000

Infectious disease	Total infectious deaths per year (approximately)
AIDS	2 600 000
Infantile respiratory infection	3 500 000
Infantile diarrhoea	2 200 000
Tuberculosis	1 500 000
Malaria	1 100 000
Measles	900 000
Neonatal tetanus	400 000
Whooping cough	350 000

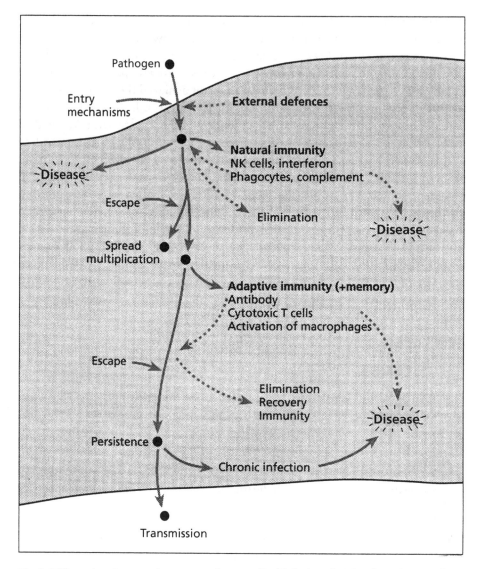

Fig. 1.4 The various stages and outcomes of a generalized infection, showing the main strategies available to the pathogen (left) and the host (right).

disease may be the result of the parasite ensuring its own spread through the tissues or its transmission to another host, and the occasional death is the price paid for this. Nevertheless, it does appear to be a reasonably safe statement that, in general, the more successful parasites are those that cause their hosts less distress.

In this book, immunity will be considered in its broadest sense, including the devices by which hosts try to keep parasites out as well as those they use against the ones that get in. You will see that these devices are very numerous and tailored to different requirements—some act fast, others are more accurate but take time; some are fairly 'broad spectrum' while others display the most exquisite specificity against individual microbial molecules. You will also see that, not surprisingly, all successful parasites, whether or not they are pathogens, have evolved counterdevices to prevent themselves being eliminated. Often these escape mechanisms are even more remarkable than those deployed by the host immune system. After all, parasites have been evolving for longer than we have, and at a vastly higher rate. However, you will perhaps be surprised to learn that, in many cases, the actual symptoms of an infectious disease are sometimes caused by the immune system itself rather than by the parasite, emphasizing the point that immune defence mechanisms are very potent, and are not absolutely guaranteed against doing damage to innocent parties such as host tissues (*immunopathology*).

You will see that this raises other very interesting questions, to which immunologists devote a lot of their time, such as: what are the limits to immunity? What regulates the activity of the immune system? How does it know which devices to use against which infection? How can it distinguish friend from foe, or in immunological parlance *self from not-self*? By bearing such questions in mind, you can sometimes see more clearly why one infectious disease takes a particular course, or another proves difficult or even impossible to get rid of. Note that the famous 'postulates' of Robert Koch (1891)* which laid down the rules for attributing a particular disease to a particular organism, did not take account of the role of the immune system and other host elements (or of multiple infections) in pathology and, though generally valid, are no longer regarded as sacrosanct.

Pursuing this idea of seeing infection from the parasite's viewpoint, it is useful to consider all infectious disease as a sort of 'obstacle course' in which the parasite's objective is to enter and survive in a host and, when appropriate, spread to another. Meanwhile the host's objective is to prevent this by all available means. Figure 1.4 is a simple 'map' of the resulting conflict, showing the main host strategies (i.e. defences) and the potential strategies for avoiding them as practised by pathogens. Most of this book consists of a description of these competing mechanisms, emphasizing that not all are equally involved, or involved at all, in every single disease, which is why different infectious diseases appear so different, just as different battles do, but also bringing out the underlying similarity. As you proceed through the book you may find it useful to refer back to this figure to check on how far along the obstacle race you have gone.

An increasingly important group of individuals comprises those whose immune system is faulty for some reason, not only because they may be more

---

*Koch's postulates state that:
1. The organism should be found in all cases of the disease, in the same location as the pathological lesions, and not in healthy individuals.
2. The organism should be grown in pure culture.
3. The culture should reproduce the disease when introduced into another susceptible host.
4. The organism should be isolated from this host and recultured.

susceptible to certain infections than the rest of us, but also because a lot has been learned from them, and from animals that have been deliberately made *immunodeficient*, about the workings of the normal system. It is true in immunology as in any other branch of biology that the best way to find out the real importance of some organ, cell, or molecule is to see what happens when it is missing, or when you remove it. The alternative approach—to assume that because two events happen together, one must be the cause of the other—is much less reliable, and immunology is full of examples where some powerful immune response turns out to be quite unrelated to the outcome of a particular infection.

In Part 3 we shall look at some applications of immunological principles, which include one of the finest achievements of all medicine, namely, *vaccination*. It is ironic that this was introduced into Europe over 200 years ago by a country physician (Jenner) at a time when neither microbiology nor immunology existed as disciplines, and was given its scientific basis 100 years later by a microbiologist (Pasteur) when immunology was thought of as a part of microbiology. We will also take a passing look at *chemotherapy*, the brainchild of a chemist (Ehrlich) who is often regarded as the first immunologist. The moral, perhaps, is that disciplines and specialties come and go according to the pace of discovery, but the study of infection and immunity remains one of the most important and fascinating in the whole of biological science.

Finally, we integrate all this knowledge in a review of the major infectious diseases of man, viewed microbiologically, immunologically, and medically, ending with a look ahead at what new problems may be awaiting us in the future.

2   Viruses

Viruses were discovered just before 1900 and used to be known as 'filterable viruses' to emphasize their small size, all but the largest being visible only in the electron microscope. It is debatable whether they should really be considered as living organisms, since they consist merely of nucleic acid wrapped in a coat of protein and depend entirely on a host cell for their metabolism and multiplication (just as 'computer viruses' need the computer's hardware before they can wreak their havoc; for once the analogy is a rather good one). But living or not, viruses are the most widespread of all pathogens, capable of infecting every species of animal from mammals down to insects, protozoa, and even bacteria, as well as plants (the well-known tobacco mosaic virus was the first virus to be transmitted experimentally, in 1876, although its nature was not understood at the time). It has been estimated that there are more species of virus than of all other creatures put together. By no means all are harmful; indeed their ability to act as 'mobile genes' is thought to have influenced the genetic make-up and evolution of higher organisms. In fact their resemblance to the genes of higher animals that can 'jump' from one chromosome to another may be a clue to their origin: many experts now believe that they are descended from bacterial *plasmids*, which are little packets of genes lying outside the bacterial chromosomes and capable of being transferred to another bacterium (see Chapters 3 and 28 for a discussion of the role of plasmids in antibiotic resistance). Another less-favoured theory is that viruses are degenerate bacteria that have given up the free-living lifestyle. Recently viruses have come to play an important role in the development of *gene therapy* because of the ease with which they can enter cells, taking in with them a selected gene to replace one missing in the recipient.

Viral structure and function

Though they vary greatly in size and complexity, viruses have certain features in common. Figure 2.1 shows the organization of a typical virus particle. Because the genome consists only of DNA or RNA, but not both, the way in which viruses replicate themselves varies from virus to virus, depending on the nature of its genome, the object in every case being to make viral proteins plus more

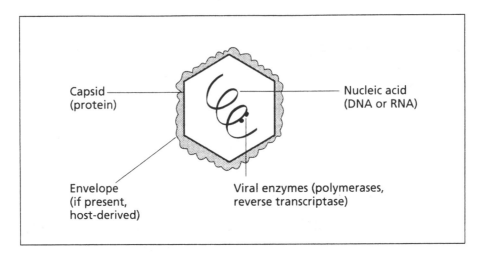

Fig. 2.1 Basic structure of a typical virus.

copies of the viral genome. DNA viruses are the simplest, since the host cell's RNA polymerase can make mRNA which can then be translated on host ribosomes to make viral proteins. RNA viruses have to provide their own RNA polymerase to make mRNA, and in the case of 'negative sense' RNA viruses an additional transcriptional step is required to make positive sense RNA. Yet another approach, used by (RNA) retroviruses, which carry the enzyme *reverse transcriptase*, is to make their own DNA which is then inserted into the host genome (Fig. 2.2). The replication of viral nucleic acid, the synthesis of viral proteins, and their assembly into new viral particles may take place in the host cell's nucleus or, less often, in the cytoplasm, depending on the virus.

A remarkable feature of most viruses is the symmetrical structure of their protein coat, built up of one or more subunits packed in a way that recalls a chemical crystal more than a form of life. Figure 2.3 illustrates two kinds of symmetry favoured by viruses. Viruses unfortunately do not lend themselves to the branched system of classification used for most animals, and are usually classified on the basis of their *nucleic acid* and whether or not they possess a lipid *envelope* outside their protein coat (Table 2.1). This envelope is acquired by the virus from the host cell in the process of making its exit—a process known as *budding*—which enables the virus to survive outside the cell sufficiently long, for example, to spread elsewhere via the bloodstream. Whether a particular virus spreads in this way or directly from one cell to its immediate neighbour has a considerable bearing on both the pattern of infection and the development of immunity. Thus an enveloped virus can leave its host cell without destroying it, while the non-enveloped sort will rupture the cell ('cytolysis'); the latter are known as *cytopathic* viruses because of their ability to damage cells and tissues, that is, cause *pathology*. Figure 2.4 illustrates these two means of spread.

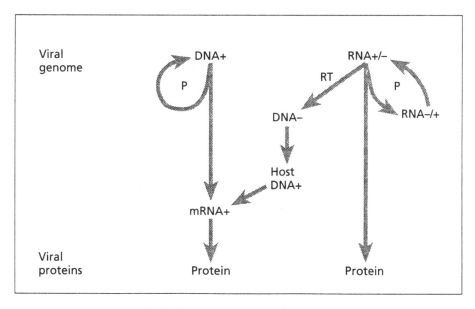

Fig. 2.2 Viruses replicate and make their proteins by several routes, depending on the nature of their genome. + and − refer to the sense of the DNA or RNA; P is polymerase, which may be host- or virus-derived; RT is reverse transcriptase, an enzyme found in retroviruses.

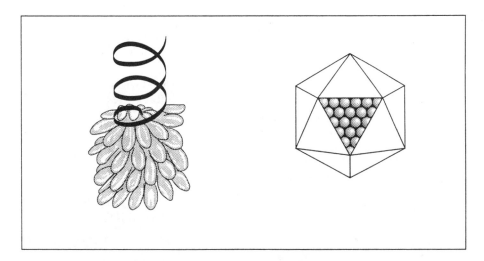

Fig. 2.3 The two most common types of viral symmetry. *Left*, helical (e.g. mumps, measles). The RNA is shown at the top and the surrounding capsid units (capsomeres) below. *Right*, icosahedral (e.g. polio). Ten of the 20 faces of the capsid are shown and 21 of the 252 capsomeres.

Having left one cell, a virus must enter another in order to multiply. Viruses are not simply taken into cells as water is, but must first attach to a *receptor* on the cell surface. Each virus has its specific receptor, usually a vital component of the cell surface—if it were not, the cell could simply shed the receptor or stop making it, and thus resist infection. Some examples of known virus–receptor pairs are

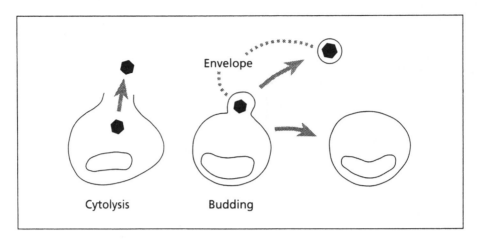

Fig. 2.4 The two methods of viral escape from the infected cell have very different effects on the cell.

Table 2.1 A simple classification of the principal viruses infecting man

	DNA	RNA
Enveloped	Herpes viruses 1, 2 3(VZV), 4(CMV) 5(EBV), 6, 7, 8	Orthomyxoviruses Influenza Paramyxoviruses Measles, mumps, Respiratory syncytial virus
	Pox viruses Smallpox	Rhabdoviruses Rabies
	Hepadna viruses Hepatitis B	Retroviruses HIV, HTLV-1
		Togaviruses Rubella
		Flaviviruses Yellow fever, dengue Hepatitis C
		Coronaviruses (colds)
		Arenaviruses Lassa fever
Non-enveloped	Adenoviruses (colds, etc.)	Picornaviruses Rhinoviruses
	Parvoviruses Papovaviruses (warts, etc.)	Enteroviruses Polio, coxsackie, hepatitis A, echo
		Reoviruses Rotavirus

Abbreviations: VZV, varicella zoster virus; CMV, cytomegalovirus; EBV, Epstein–Barr virus; HIV, human immunodeficiency virus; HTLV, human T-lymphotropic virus.

Table 2.2 For some viruses, the cell-surface receptor required for attachment and subsequent entry is known, but for many others it remains to be discovered

Virus	Receptor
Epstein–Barr	B cell complement receptor CR2
HIV	T cell, macrophage CD4, CCR5, CXCR4
Rhinovirus	Adhesion molecule ICAM-1
Rabies	Acetylcholine receptor
Vaccinia	Epidermal growth factor receptor
Influenza	Neuraminic acid (also on red cells)
Reovirus	β adrenergic hormone receptor
Poliovirus	Lipoprotein?
Echo, coxsackie	CD55/DAF
Measles	CD46

shown in Table 2.2. It is the distribution of these receptor molecules on host cells that largely determines the cell-preference (or *tropism*) of individual viruses. For example, the human immunodeficiency virus (HIV) infects mainly T lymphocytes and macrophages because only they carry a surface molecule known as CD4 (see Appendix 3), while EBV infects B lymphocytes carrying the complement receptor CR2.

Infection of a cell by a virus can have one of several effects. Many viruses cause no harm or disease whatever. But as mentioned earlier, the cell may be lysed as the viral particles burst out and spread elsewhere—a *lytic* infection. Eventually, if host immunity operates effectively, the virus-infected cell may be killed by the host, leading to interruption of the virus cycle and cure of the infection. Not all viruses are got rid of so easily. They may persist in the cell without damaging it, giving rise to the *carrier* state, in which an apparently cured patient can still be infectious to others. Or they may survive in a non-infectious form that can become reactivated to cause a second infection; this is called *latency*. Table 2.3 lists some well-known examples of these different outcomes.

Viruses and cancer

Finally, the viral DNA (or DNA copied from viral RNA) may become integrated into host DNA, with effects on the control of cell growth that can in some cases lead to *transformation*, in other words a tumour. However, integration does not always lead to transformation, nor is it essential for tumour formation. The association of viruses with tumours in animals was first suspected 90 years ago but

Table 2.3 Viral infection can lead to several different outcomes for the infected cell

Lysis (cytopathic)	Persistence (carrier state)	Latency (reactivation)	Transformation	
			Benign	Malignant
Adenovirus	Hepatitis B	Herpesviruses (HSV; VZV; CMV)	Warts	Hepatitis B (liver cancer)
Influenza	EB virus			
Poliovirus				EB virus (Burkitt's lymphoma)

Abbreviations: HSV, herpes simplex virus; VZV, varicella zoster virus; CMV, cytomegalovirus.

Table 2.4 Landmarks in the understanding of tumour viruses

1908	Bang, Ellerman	Chicken leukaemia transmitted by filtrable particle
1911	Rous	Chicken sarcoma ″ ″ ″ ″
1930	Shope	Rabbit skin tumours ″ ″ ″ ″
1936	Bittner	Mouse breast cancer transmitted by milk factor
1962	Burkitt	Human lymphoma due to infection?
1964	Epstein, Barr	Virus extracted from Burkitt's lymphoma
1977	Blumberg	Liver carcinoma due to hepatitis B virus
1980	Gallo	HTLV-1 causes T cell leukaemia
1994	Chang, Moore	HHV-8 causes Kaposi's sarcoma; some HPV types cause cervical and skin cancer

Abbreviations: HTLV, human T-lymphotropic virus; HPV, human papilloma virus.

only in the 1960s was a virus (EBV) shown convincingly to be associated with a human tumour (Burkitt's lymphoma). Table 2.4 illustrates some key dates in the gradual unfolding of the virus–cancer link. The mechanism by which viruses push cells into the uncontrolled growth characteristic of tumours appears to involve *oncogenes*, of either viral or host origin. In some cases these genes code for growth factor receptors on the cell surface, in other cases the virus inhibits the cell's tumour suppressor genes or the normal process of cell suicide (apoptosis), and sometimes other factors come in. One of the most complex pathways is that by which heavy EBV infection, malaria infection, and the translocation of the cellular oncogene c-myc to a site active in B lymphocytes, all come together to induce the B-cell tumour known as Burkitt's lymphoma.

Spread and control

As well as replicating themselves in the host, most viruses need to spread to another host, since the original host may either die or eliminate the infection (how this happens will be described in later chapters). The main routes of spread are listed in Table 2.5. Meanwhile, in order to survive long enough to spread to another host, viruses may often need to escape the attentions of the immune system. How they do this is described in detail in Chapters 12 and 21 where you will see that some of their strategies are very sophisticated, such as repeatedly changing their surface molecules or switching off immune responses. A special category of viruses is those that cause disease only when the immune system is deficient in some way; these are called opportunists, and *opportunistic infection* is one of

Table 2.5 The principal routes of viral spread

Route	Examples
Skin contact	HPV (warts)
Respiratory	Cold viruses, influenza, measles, mumps, rubella
Faecal–oral	Polio; echo; coxsackie; hepatitis A; rotavirus
Milk	HIV, HTLV-1, CMV
Transplacental	Rubella, CMV, HIV
Sexually	Herpes 1, 2; HIV; HPV; hepatitis B
Insect vector	Yellow fever; dengue
Animal bite	Rabies

Abbreviations: HPV, human papilloma virus; HIV, human immunodeficiency virus; HTLV, human T-lymphotropic virus; CMV, cytomegalovirus.

Table 2.6 Some zoonotic viruses

Virus	Animal reservoir
Influenza	Birds; pigs; horses
Rabies	Bats; dogs; foxes
Lassa, Hanta viruses	Rodents
Ebola; Marburg viruses	Monkeys
HIV 1; 2	Chimpanzees; monkeys
Newcastle disease	Poultry
West Nile virus	Birds

the main problems in patients with, for example, AIDS. How individual viruses and the immune system interact to set the pattern of disease is described in Chapter 30.

The pattern of viral disease has been radically altered by the introduction of *vaccines*. Many of the really successful vaccines are against viruses, and one disease—smallpox—has been completely eliminated (1980). It is hoped that several other viruses, such as polio and measles, will follow. This is just as well because the development of antiviral drugs still has far to go. Further details are given in Chapters 27 and 28. Nevertheless there are unfortunately a number of viruses that at present do not seem promising candidates for vaccines. In addition, apparently 'new' viruses crop up from time to time, usually by spreading from an animal in which they are well adapted to humans in which they are not; these *zoonoses* include some of the most frightening and acutely fatal of all virus diseases (Table 2.6 and Chapter 35).

3 Bacteria

With the bacteria, we enter the world of cellular organisms, capable of fully independent existence and within range of the ordinary light microscope. Bacteria were almost certainly the first truly living things on our planet, representing a high degree of organization within a single cell. Some are parasitic, but the majority live free in soil, water, etc., while some can live free or as parasites as it suits them. However, bacteria differ fundamentally from all other cellular organisms, whether unicellular like the fungi and protozoa or multicellular like worms (and man), in that they are *procaryotic* rather than *eucaryotic*. The distinction between these two forms of cellular organization is important to the understanding of how they respond to the immune system, and also, as Chapter 28 will show, to therapeutic drugs. The principal features of the two types of cell are illustrated in Fig. 3.1.

Classification: the cell wall

One part of the bacterium with a special significance for both disease and immunity is the *cell wall*, and bacterial classification starts with the distinction between three types of cell wall that vary greatly in their structure (Fig. 3.2). Conveniently for microbiologists, a simple iodine/crystal violet-based technique, the Gram stain, identifies two fundamentally different types: *Gram-positive* (stained), with a thick sugar amino-acid polymer (peptidoglycan) outside a single cell membrane, and *Gram-negative* (unstained) with a thinner peptidoglycan layer between two cell membranes. A third group, the mycobacteria, have waxy outer layers that resist the Gram stain and can be visualized using a fuchsin-based stain (Ziehl–Neelsen or 'ZN'). Their tough wall has earned them the name 'acid fast bacilli' (AFB).

The cell wall has a considerable influence on bacterial survival; thus peptidoglycan is resistant to digestion by bile but sensitive to the enzyme *lysozyme* (and also to penicillin; see Chapter 28), while the waxy mycolic acids of mycobacteria enhance long-term survival in dry conditions. Other external features of some bacteria are the capsule (see below) and long processes that facilitate motility (flagella) or attachment to host cells (pili).

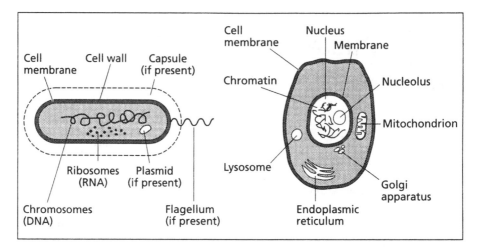

Fig. 3.1 Procaryotic and eucaryotic cells compared. *Left*, a typical (procaryotic) bacterium. *Right*, a typical eucaryotic cell.

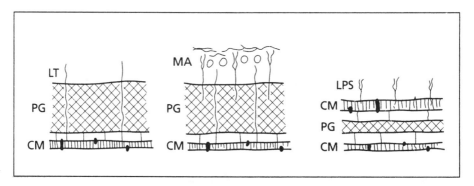

Fig. 3.2 Three types of bacterial cell wall, showing the single or double cell membrane (CM). *Left*, Gram-positive (e.g. *Staphylococcus*); the exposed peptidoglycan (PG) is accessible to host lysosomal enzymes; LT, lipoteichoic acid. *Centre*, mycobacterium (e.g. *M. tuberculosis*); the surface coat of the lipid mycolic acid (MA) confers resistance to acid, alcohol, and many immune killing mechanisms. *Right*, Gram-negative (e.g. salmonella); the lipopolysaccharide (LPS) inserted in the outer cell membrane is an important virulence factor.

Beyond this level, bacteria are classified according to shape into the roughly spherical *cocci* and the long thin *rods*, plus an assorted group of 'atypical' bacteria. Further subdivisions are made on the basis of growth requirements, possession of particular surface molecules or *antigens* (a term you will meet when we discuss antibody in Chapter 16), and the sequences of their proteins and nucleic acids; ribosomal RNA is used increasingly as a reliable index of evolutionary relationships between organisms, all the way from bacteria to mammals. Table 3.1 lists the main bacteria of importance in human and animal disease. Some of these, like some of the viruses, are opportunists.

Table 3.1 The medically important bacteria

	Gram-positive	Gram-negative

Cocci (spherical)	Staphylococci
	Streptococci
		Neisseria
		  Meningococcus
		  Gonococcus

Bacilli (rod-shaped)	*Bacillus anthracis*	Enteric

	Clostridium
	  tetani
	  perfringens
	  botulinum
		Salmonella
		Shigella
		Escherichia
		Yersinia

	Corynebacterium *diphtheriae*	*Pseudomonas*
	Listeria	*Vibrio* *cholerae*
		Campylobacter
		Helicobacter

	*Mycobacterium
	  tuberculosis
	  leprae
		Brucella

		Haemophilus
		Bordetella
		Legionella
		Bacteroides
Filamentous	Actinomycetes	

Spiral		*Spirochaetes
		  Treponema
		  Leptospira
		  Borrelia

Obligate intracellular		*Chlamydiae *Rickettsiae
Lacking cell walls	*Mycoplasma	

Those in the group below the line are often referred to as 'atypical' (see text). Note that the Gram-positive cocci and the Gram-negative rods are responsible for the majority of severe bacterial disease. The asterisked organisms (*) are not normally identified by the Gram stain, but share characteristics of the Gram-positive or Gram-negative groups as shown.

Unlike eucaryotic cells, bacteria have no clear-cut nuclei, their DNA being in the form of a single, usually circular, chromosome without introns. A system of repressor, inducer, and co-repressor molecules ensures economical regulation of the genes coding for bacterial enzymes appropriate to the available substrates. Further DNA may be present in the form of small circular *plasmids*, which carry genes for adaptive functions such as toxin production and antibiotic resistance (see below). Sometimes a plasmid is large enough to be considered as a second chromosome (e.g. in *Vibrio cholerae*); indeed it is thought that eucaryotic chromosomes may have evolved from plasmids that became segregated into nuclei.

Metabolism

Parasitic bacteria, unlike plants and some free-living bacteria, lack chlorophyll and cannot obtain energy from photosynthesis. Instead, they use various inorganic molecules and glucose, from which they derive energy by glycolysis (fermentation); some can go further and use oxygen (respiration). The *mitochondria* of higher animals are believed to have originated from bacteria that were taken up and used by early eucaryotes to enable them to respire (in a similar way, the *plant* cell probably evolved from the uptake of photosynthetic bacteria). This distinction between aerobic and anaerobic bacteria shows up in certain infections. For example the aerobic tubercle bacillus grows well in the (well-oxygenated) lungs, while the anaerobic clostridia that cause tetanus and gas gangrene flourish in the oxygen-starved environment of deep wounds.

Atypical bacteria

Not all bacteria fit neatly into the foregoing classification. *Spirochaetes* are unusual in being helically coiled, highly motile, and resistant to Gram-staining. *Actinomycetes* are filamentous, and were formerly considered to be fungi. Poised between viruses and typical bacteria are the *Rickettsiae* and *Chlamydiae*. Like bacteria they have both DNA and RNA, but like viruses they are obligate intracellular parasites because they lack some of the biosynthetic pathways for independent existence. *Mycoplasmas*, on the other hand, can survive extracellularly, despite their lack of a cell wall. Table 3.2 lists those important as human pathogens; see Chapter 31 for further details.

Genetics and reproduction

Bacterial replication normally occurs by simple binary fission and may be extremely fast (every 20 minutes for some staphylococci) or very slow (around 2 weeks for the leprosy bacillus); for comparison, a time of 24 hours would be considered rapid for mammalian cells. As with all dividing cells, bacteria can acquire variations by *mutations* in their DNA, some of which can be useful to them, for example if they confer resistance to a therapeutic drug or a host defence mechanism. However, bacteria can also vary their genome more extensively by taking in DNA from other bacteria, a process known as *lateral gene transfer*, which can take several forms, including transformation, transduction by viruses known as

Table 3.2 The major pathogenic atypical bacteria

Group	Examples	Human disease
Actinomycetes	*Antinomyces israelii*	Actinomycosis
Spirochaetes	*Treponema pallidum*	Syphilis
	Leptospira interrogans	Weil's disease
	Borrelia recurrentis	Relapsing fever
	B. burgdorferi	Lyme disease
Rickettsiae	*Rickettsia typhi*	Typhus
	Coxiella burnetii	Q fever
Chlamydiae	*Chlamydia trachomatis*	Trachoma
	C. psittaci	Psittacosis
Mycoplasma	*M. pneumoniae*	Atypical pneumonia

bacteriophages, recombination, and a process of *conjugation* between two bacteria that comes close to resembling the sexual process of higher animals (Fig. 3.3). Sometimes it is a *plasmid* that is transferred; plasmids code for a number of proteins useful to the bacteria such as toxins, adhesion molecules, and resistance factors (collectively known as *virulence factors*; see Chapter 8). Another method for bringing about rapid changes in genes is *phase variation*, by which mispairing of repeat sequences causes the synthesis of important proteins to be switched on or off. These strategies, combined with rapid replication, frequently allow bacteria to keep 'one jump ahead' of their environment; one topical example of this is the continuous emergence of staphylococci resistant to many or even all antibiotics—the dreaded 'hospital staphs' (see Chapter 28). Conversely, genes that are no longer required may be rendered non-functional and eventually lost, a process known as *gene decay*; for example bacteria adapted to intracellular existence have smaller genomes than free-living ones, since they can use some host biosynthetic pathways.

Some bacteria can halt their growth altogether under adverse conditions and form *spores*, which can lie dormant for years until the conditions for growth reappear. This is how, for example, tetanus bacilli are able to survive in the soil; and cause rapid infections if they get into a wound.

Disease and immunity

Bacteria do not always cause disease, in fact the intestine of a healthy adult contains about 10^{14} bacteria (more as you move down the bowel) with perhaps another 10^{12} on the skin. The value of this 'normal flora' has been the subject of

	Transformation	**Transduction**	**Conjugation**
Form of DNA transferred	Naked (small pieces)	In bacteriophage	In plasmid
Transfer / Integration	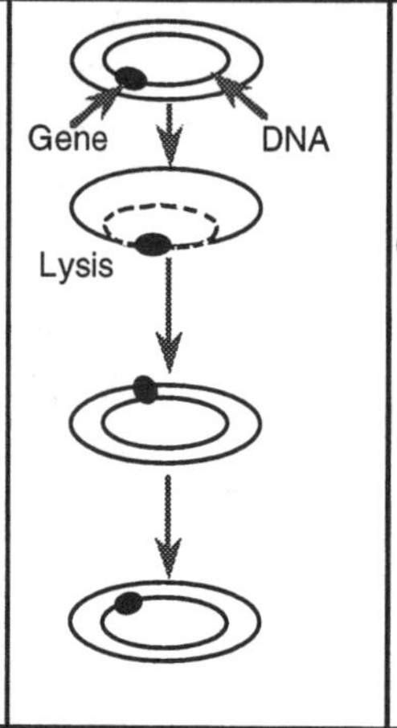 Gene DNA / Lysis	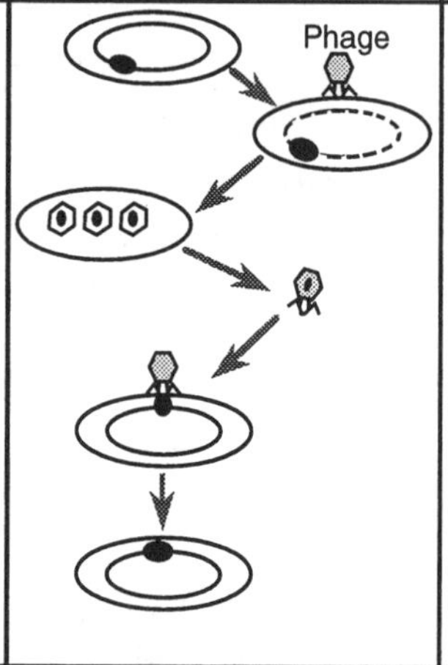 Phage	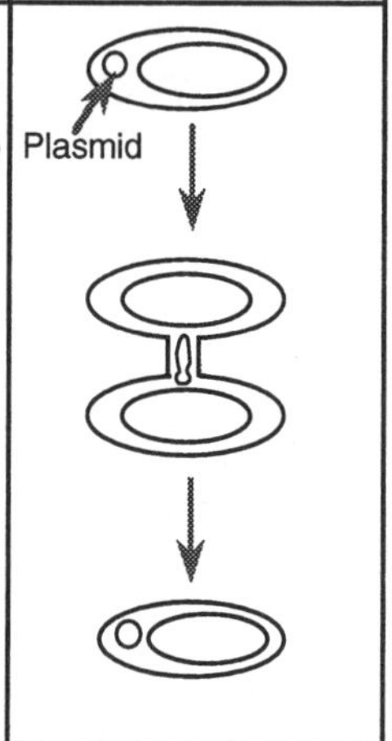 Plasmid
Example	'Competent' strains only eg *S. pneumoniae*	Many toxin genes	Antibiotic resistant genes

Fig. 3.3 Bacteria can acquire new genes in several ways.

much argument, but it does appear that interfering with it can be dangerous; for example, by allowing other more harmful organisms to establish themselves. However, some bacteria do unfortunately cause very severe disease, as will be described in Chapter 8. Gastrointestinal disease, much of it bacterial, is a major infective cause of death worldwide, with tuberculosis not far behind (see Table 1.2).

Like all parasites, bacteria have evolved numerous mechanisms for avoiding elimination by the immune system. Strategies of particular relevance to bacteria include the production of a *capsule*—a slimy polysaccharide coat that covers the cell wall—various ways of inhibiting phagocytic cells, and other ingenious devices to be described later (Chapters 9, 12, and 21). As a result, bacteria are responsible for several chronic infections, for example, tuberculosis, leprosy, and brucellosis. Another common feature of bacteria is the production of *toxins*, which can cause some of the most acute and serious diseases, including tetanus, cholera, and gas gangrene. Toxins will be discussed in detail in Chapter 8, and the immunology of particular bacterial diseases in Chapter 31.

Table 3.3 Some zoonotic bacterial infections

Bacterium	Animal reservoir	Disease
Mycobacterium bovis	Cattle	Tuberculosis
Mycobacterium avium	Birds	Pneumonia
Leptospira spp.	Horse, cattle, dog	Weil's disease
Clostridium tetani	Horse, sheep, cattle	Tetanus
Brucella spp.	Cattle, goat, dog	Brucellosis
Borrelia spp.	Deer	Lyme disease
E. coli (EHEC)	Farm animals (meat, milk)	Food poisoning
Salmonella spp.	" " eggs	" "
Campylobacter spp.	" "	" "
Yersinia pestis	Rat	Plague
Bacillus anthracis	Farm animals	Anthrax

As with viruses, many bacteria can be acquired from animals, in which they may be better adapted and so less pathogenic (see Table 3.3).

Antibacterial vaccines and drugs

With respect to therapy, the situation with bacteria is almost the opposite of that with viruses. The control of bacterial disease by *antibiotics* has been one of the twentieth century's success stories, though we are not nearly as optimistic as we were (see 'hospital staphs', above). On the other hand, there are not many really good bacterial *vaccines* (Chapter 27 explains why this is) and certainly very few bacterial diseases that look like candidates for elimination. Since the eucaryotic pathogens, described in the next three chapters, are generally commoner in tropical countries, it seems likely that in the years to come bacteria will be the major cause of infectious disease in the developed world.

Useful bacteria

We should not forget the remarkable number of ways in which bacteria, far from being pathogenic, are useful and even essential to humans and animals. Table 3.4 lists a few of these useful functions.

Table 3.4 Some useful functions of bacteria

Soil	Nitrogen fixation; biodegradation
Cattle rumen	Digestion
Human intestine ('normal flora')	Compete for space with pathogens (Some) vitamin synthesis
Dairy industry	Fermentation (e.g. cheese, yoghurt)
Energy industry	Methane ('natural gas'); recycling of waste
Pharmaceutical industry	Production of enzymes, antibiotics
Biotechnology	Plasmids as vectors

4   Fungi

When one thinks of mushrooms and toadstools, the idea of a fungus parasitic on humans seems rather improbable, but most fungi are not this large, existing as single cells (yeasts) or slender filaments (moulds), while some exist as a mixture of both (dimorphic). Out of a total of some 70 000 species, about 300 are parasites of animals, and of these a few (shown in Table 4.1) are of major importance as human pathogens.

Structure and morphology

Unlike bacteria, fungi are *eucaryotes*, with a basic cell design very similar to our own but with a complex cell wall stiffened by the addition of polysaccharides such as chitin, glucans, and mannans. Another difference is that in most cases the plasma membrane contains ergosterol in place of cholesterol (Fig. 4.1).

Yeasts and moulds differ mainly in their means of reproduction—a process of *budding* in yeasts and *apical extension* in moulds (Fig. 4.2). Dimorphic fungi behave as moulds at environmental temperatures but switch to the yeast form at body temperature. Most fungi are acquired from soil or decaying plants via inhalation of spores or from animals (e.g. *Microsporum* from cats and dogs; *Cryptococcus* from bird droppings) or other humans (e.g. *Trichophyton*).

In size, the single-celled fungi lie between bacteria and mammalian cells, and are therefore small enough to be taken in by host phagocytes (for a description of these important host defence cells, see Chapter 11) in which they sometimes manage to survive. This has the result that some fungal diseases or *mycoses* (e.g. histoplasmosis) closely resemble diseases caused by bacteria with a similar lifestyle (e.g. the tubercle bacillus), though the organisms themselves are totally different in structure and physiology. When you consider that some protozoa behave similarly, you will appreciate that the precise taxonomic status of the microbe is not all that matters in pathogenesis; its habitat in the body, the immunity it evokes, and how it escapes this are quite as important in dictating the outcome. Indeed, one microorganism, *Pneumocystis carinii*, a major cause of disease in immunodeficient patients (that is, an opportunist), has recently had to be

Table 4.1 The principal medically important fungi

	Yeasts	Dimorphic	Filamentous
Superficial infection	*Candida*	*Malassezia*	*Microsporum*
			Trichophyton
Subcutaneous		*Sporothrix*	*Madurella*
Systemic dissemination	**Cryptococcus*	*Histoplasma*	**Aspergillus*
	*Candida	*Blastomyces*	**Zygomyces*
	†Pneumocystis	*Coccidioides*	**Fusarium*
		Paracoccidioides	

* Opportunists, i.e. pathogenic only in immunodeficient individuals.
† A single-celled opportunist, but taxonomic status uncertain.

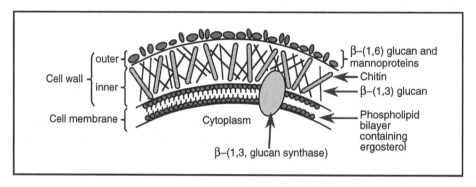

Fig. 4.1 The typical structure of the fungal cell wall.

reclassified on the basis of its ribosomal RNA as a fungus, having hitherto been accepted as a protozoan!

The eucaryotic parasites pose particular problems to the host because their cells resemble those of the host much more closely than bacteria (or indeed viruses) do. When we come to consider the way in which the immune system recognizes the presence of an invading microbe, you will appreciate why fungi, protozoa, and worms are usually hard to get rid of and, by the same token, hard to eliminate by chemotherapy.

Cutaneous and superficial mycoses

Collectively known as dermatophytes, these fungi grow on skin, nails, and hair. *Trichophyton* and *Microsporum* spp. cause tinea (capitis, corporis: ringworm; pedis: athlete's foot). *Malasezzia* causes pityriasis. The yeast *Candida albicans* is a normal commensal of the gut and moist skin sites, but can overgrow in the

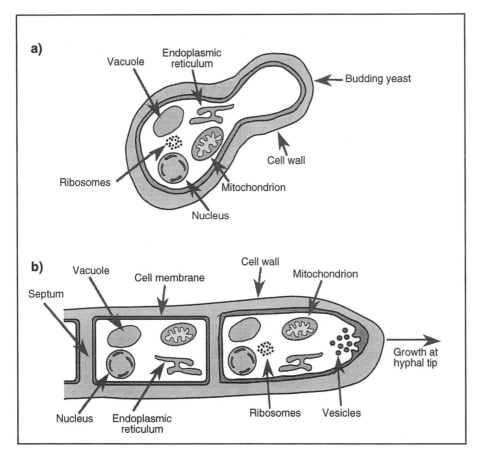

Fig. 4.2 Reproduction in fungi. (a) A budding yeast cell; (b) the growing tip of a filamentous mould.

mouth and vagina, causing thrush, particularly following long-term antibiotic treatment which disturbs the normal bacterial flora.

Subcutaneous mycoses

Sporothrix, common in gardeners, causes the ulcerating nodules of sporotrichosis. *Madurella* causes the swollen and destructive lesions of Madura foot.

Systemic mycoses

Mostly acquired by inhalation of spores, *Histoplasma*, *Blastomyces*, *Coccidioides*, and *Paracoccidioides* are a frequent cause of pneumonia in parts of

Central America. In immunocompromised patients (see Chapters 14, 24, and 25 for a discussion of the causes of immunodeficiency) these infections can become widely disseminated and may be fatal. The same is true for a number of normally less pathogenic fungi, notably *Aspergillus*, *Cryptococcus*, *Candida*, and *Pneumocystis*. What this teaches us about the role of the immune system is discussed in Chapter 32.

Useful fungi

Yeasts, of course, have their beneficial side too, an obvious example being the ability of *Saccharomyces* spp. in aerobic conditions to convert sugars into CO_2 (which helps bread dough to rise) and, in anaerobic conditions, alcohol (the basis of the wine and beer industry). Recently, yeasts have proved to be good cells in which to insert foreign genes so as to manufacture large amounts of a pure protein; the current hepatitis B vaccine is made in this way. And of course one should not forget that penicillin was originally obtained from the mould *Penicillium notatum*.

5 Protozoa

The protozoa (the name means 'first animals') are single-celled eucaryotes of amazing diversity and sophistication. The vast majority live free, employing a range of special structures for moving, adhering, killing other organisms, etc., but a few are parasites of man or domestic animals and some of these are major pathogens. Their medical importance is heightened by the fact that they are very successful as parasites, hard for the immune system to dislodge, and hard to design effective drugs against. Most of the really severe protozoal diseases are restricted to the tropics because they depend on an insect or other *vector* and often an *animal reservoir* which is only found there.

Like bacteria and fungi, protozoa can be extracellular or intracellular parasites, as is shown in Table 5.1 together with an indication of how they are generally classified. Their impact on the affected areas can be judged from Table 5.2. One of them, the malaria parasite, has a life cycle of remarkable complexity (see below), but this is unusual, and most protozoa have relatively simple life cycles.

As might be predicted from their success as parasites, protozoa have very well-developed mechanisms for eluding the immune system of their hosts, often by varying their antigens and/or suppressing immunity; how these affect the course of disease will be described in the last section of this book (Chapter 33). Some, such as *Toxoplasma*, are opportunists, normally harmless but pathogenic in those who are immunodeficient. It seems likely that, with the increasing numbers of immunodeficient individuals (see Chapters 24 and 25), the difficulty in making effective protozoal vaccines (see Chapter 27), the development of drug resistance (see Chapter 28), and the prospect of climate changes through global warming, protozoa will become more important as human pathogens.

Malaria

The malaria parasite, *Plasmodium*, has a life cycle whose origin almost defies imagination, with successive stages in the mosquito gut and salivary glands, via a mosquito bite to human blood, the liver, the blood again, with a repeating ('*asexual*') cycle through the red cell, and thence via another bite back to the mosquito (Fig. 5.1). An unusual feature is the development in the host red cell of

Table 5.1 The protozoa of medical significance

Means of spread	Habitat	
	Extracellular	Intracellular
Insect-borne*	African trypanosome (blood)	*Plasmodium* (liver, red cell) *Leishmania* (macrophage) S. American trypanosome (macrophage; muscle; nerve)
Water-borne or other routes	Amoeba (gut) *Giardia* (gut) †*Cryptosporidium* (gut) *Isospora* (gut) *Trichomonas* (urogenital)	†*Toxoplasma* (macrophage)

* The protozoa carried by insect vectors are mainly confined to the tropics by the distribution of the vectors. † *Toxoplasma* and *Cryptosporidium* are important opportunists.

Table 5.2 Approximate annual incidence and mortality for the major protozoal diseases

Disease	Incidence	Mortality
Giardiasis	500 000 000	—
Malaria	300 000 000	1 100 000
Trichomoniasis	180 000 000	—
Toxoplasmosis	100 000 000	250 000 (in AIDS)
Amoebiasis	500 000	50 000
Leishmaniasis	2 000 000	50 000
Trypanosomiasis		
African	500 000	400 000?
S. American	300 000	50 000

male and female gametes, which fuse to complete the *sexual* stage in the mosquito. The advantage to the parasite is rapid reassortment of genes, with the slight disadvantage that the host is not infectious at all times. From the host's point of view, this complex cycle means that a confusing sequence of different *antigens* is presented to the immune system, further complicated by the fact that many of them are highly polymorphic. The many species of *Plasmodium* that infect animals and birds are not infective for man; thus there is no animal reservoir for human malaria.

Four species of *Plasmodium* infect man, each with slightly different characteristics (Table 5.3). In terms of mortality, *P. falciparum* (malignant tertian) is by far the most important, being responsible for at least a million deaths per year. These

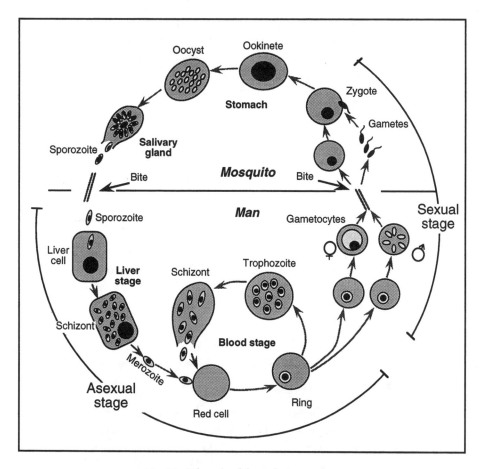

Fig. 5.1 Life cycle of the malaria parasite.

Table 5.3 The malaria parasites of man

Species	Liver stage	Blood cycle and fever peaks	Disease features
P. falciparum	6–14 days	48 hr ('tertian')	Major complications (see text); may be fatal
P. vivax	12–17 days (with relapses)	48 hr	Seldom fatal
P. malariae	13–40 days	72 hr ('quartan')	Nephrotic syndrome
P. ovale	9–18 days	50 hr	

result chiefly from *anaemia* and *cerebral malaria*, the latter being associated with the phenomenon of *sequestration*, in which parasitized red cells become attached to the vascular endothelium in the brain and other organs. Other complications include glomerulonephritis, hypoglycaemia, and pulmonary oedema. *P. vivax* does not show sequestration and complications are few, though the fever can be intense and debilitating. For further details see Chapter 33.

Leishmania

Transmitted by the bite of the sandfly, the *Leishmania* parasite is taken up by macrophages where it survives and replicates as an *amastigote* ('no tail'), settling either in the skin (cutaneous) or the spleen and liver (visceral) depending on the species (see Table 5.4). In the insect vector the flagellate *promastigote* develops in the gut for reinfection of the human host (Fig. 5.2). The cutaneous disease runs a chronic course with eventual healing, but visceral leishmaniasis can be fatal, with massive splenomegaly and liver failure. Dogs and rodents are the main reservoir of infection.

Trypanosomes

Trypanosomes belong to the same order as *Leishmania* and resemble them in appearance (Fig. 5.2). The species of *Trypanosoma* infecting man differ in their geographical distribution, vector and life cycle (Table 5.5).

Table 5.4 The principal species of *Leishmania* infecting man

Species	Areas affected	Disease pattern
L. donovani	Old World (Africa, India, Middle East)	visceral
L. infantum	"	"
L. major	"	cutaneous
L. tropica	"	"
L. aethiopica	"	"
L. mexicana	New World (Central and South America)	"
L. braziliensis	"	"
L. peruviana	"	"
L. venezuelensis	"	"
L. chagasi	"	visceral

Table 5.5 The human trypanosomes

Species	Areas affected	Vector	Disease pattern
T. brucei gambiense	West Africa	Tsetse fly	Parasite free in blood: sleeping sickness
T. brucei rhodesiense	East Africa	"	" "
T. cruzi	S. America	Reduviid bug	Macrophages; heart Chagas' disease

Stage		Leishmania	*T. brucei*	*T. cruzi*
Insect form (promastigote)	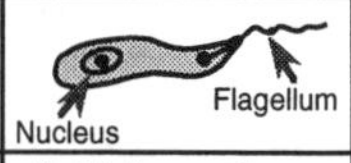 Nucleus Flagellum	Sandfly	Tsetse fly	Reduviid bug
Blood form (trypomastigote)	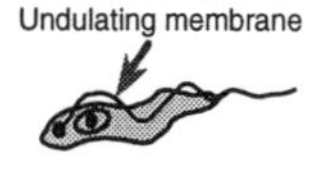 Undulating membrane	—	Free in blood	Free in blood (brief)
Intracellular/tissue form (amastigote)	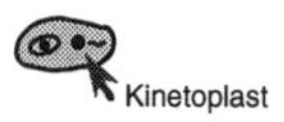 Kinetoplast	Host macrophage	Choroid plexus	Heart, CNS

Fig. 5.2 *Leishmania* and *Trypanosoma* compared.

African trypanosomes

T. brucei is unusual in living and multiplying free in the blood of its mammalian hosts, which include man and many species of cattle. This lifestyle necessitates sophisticated immune evasion strategies, as described in Chapter 21. Involvement of the CNS leads to the characteristic coma of *sleeping sickness* (see Chapter 33).

South American trypanosome

T. cruzi somewhat resembles *Leishmania* in being predominantly an intracellular parasite, after a brief blood stage (Fig. 5.2). Infection of cardiac muscle and the ganglia of the autonomic nervous system lead to chronic heart failure and dilated organs (megaoesophagus, megacolon), respectively.

Toxoplasma

Toxoplasma gondii, an intracellular parasite, common in both farm and domestic animals (particularly cats), causes symptomless infection of up to 50% of human populations, who acquire it through contaminated water, food, or faeces. The parasite can survive in the form of cysts, which can be reactivated if the host becomes immunodeficient (see Chapters 25 and 33). An active infection can be transmitted from mother to fetus via the placenta, leading to fetal damage, particularly to the brain and eye, or death.

Amoeba

Entamoeba histolytica is the cause of the well-known amoebic dysentery and occasionally of abscesses in brain, liver, and lung. The cyst form is acquired via contaminated water and develops into trophozoites in the intestine (Fig. 5.3).

Giardia

Giardia lamblia has a similar life cycle to that of *Entamoeba*, but its effects are normally limited to the intestine.

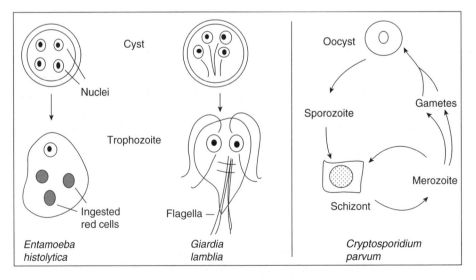

Fig. 5.3 Water-borne intestinal parasites of man.

Cryptosporidium; *Isospora*

Cryptosporidium parvum has a more complex life cycle, which includes a sexual stage (Fig. 5.3). Like *Toxoplasma*, it is an important opportunist in immunodeficient patients, particularly those with AIDS (as is the rather similar *Isospora belli*), but also causes outbreaks of diarrhoea in otherwise healthy individuals following breakdown of water purification procedures.

Trichomonas

Trichomonas vaginalis is a sexually transmitted parasite of the vagina and urethra and a common cause of vaginitis and occasionally urethritis.

6 Helminths (worms)

Worms represent the limit as far as parasite size is concerned, some of the largest ones being almost as long as their hosts (though fortunately not as bulky!). The vast majority are free living, and only three classes of worm include pathogens of man; these are listed in Table 6.1.

Worms are unlike other parasites in several respects. To begin with, they are of course *multicellular* animals, with well-developed organs and usually very tough outer coats, which makes them virtually impossible for the immune system to dislodge. However, they do induce vigorous immune responses, with an unusual emphasis on eosinophils and IgE antibody (see Chapter 16). Another difference is that with a few exceptions they do not replicate within their human host, but either free or in another host (insect, snail, etc.). From the human point of view, this means that a single worm, once acquired, remains a single worm, rather than multiplying into thousands or millions like viruses, bacteria, or protozoa. Thus the final weight of infection is directly proportional to the original number of infecting organisms (though they may increase substantially in size). This in turn has important effects on the design of preventive measures.

Although their sheer size makes worms difficult to get rid of, they also have some very sophisticated mechanisms for eluding the immune system. A striking example is the blood fluke *Schistosoma*, which manages to camouflage itself by picking up a surface coating of molecules from the blood of the host (see Chapter 21). Because they represent a huge amount of foreign material yet survive for long periods (years in some cases), parasitic worms represent some of the largest sustained challenges to the immune system. Unfortunately, a large sustained challenge frequently leads to overstimulation of the system, with harmful effects to the host. This is called *immunopathology*, and will be discussed in Chapters 22 and 34. Here, three examples of it may be quoted—the lymphoedema of the limbs caused by prolonged responses to the filarial worm *Wuchereria bancrofti*, leading to the terrible deformities of elephantiasis, the river blindness caused by another filarial worm *Onchocerca volvulus* which unfortunately likes to visit the eye, and the potentially fatal liver cirrhosis caused by the eggs of *Schistosoma mansoni*. Not only in numbers, but also in terms of prolonged human suffering, worms must rank as the most unwelcome parasites of all (Table 6.2).

Table 6.1 The major helminths of medical significance

Means of spread	Roundworms (nematodes)	Tapeworms (cestodes)	Flukes (trematodes)

Intermediate host	Filariae
	    Onchocerca (fly)
	    Wuchereria
	        (mosquito)
	    Brugia (mosquito)
	    Loa loa (fly)
			Schistosoma (snail)
			Paragonimus (crab)
			Clonorchis (fish)

Food, water, or other	*Ascaris* Hookworm *Toxocara* *Trichinella* *Strongyloides*	*Taenia* *Echinococcus* ('hydatid')	

* Mainly important as an opportunist.

Table 6.2 Worldwide prevalence of the major helminth infections

Nematodes	
Filarial	150 000 000
Intestinal	4 200 000 000
Tapeworms	175 000 000
Flukes	
Blood	200 000 000
Lung	20 000 000
Intestinal	200 000
Liver	20 000 000

Schistosomes and other flukes

Three species of the blood fluke *Schistosoma* are important human pathogens, with a worldwide distribution (Table 6.3) and complex life cycles involving an aquatic snail intermediate host (Fig. 6.1).

Schistosomiasis (also known as bilharzia) probably originated in the Nile valley, and has been identified in Egyptian mummies. Other flukes causing less serious disease include the gut flukes *Metagonimus* and *Heterophyes*, and humans may be infected by the sheep liver fluke *Fasciola* and the intestinal fluke *Fasciolopsis*.

The lung fluke *Paragonimus westermanii* has a life cycle similar to that of the schistosomes but more complex, involving two aquatic vectors—snail and

Table 6.3 Major characteristics of the human blood flukes

Species	Geographical distribution	Disease features
S. mansoni	Africa; Middle East; S. America	Dermatitis ('swimmer's itch') Abdominal pain; diarrhoea Eggs in liver → portal fibrosis → portal hypertension → haematemesis Eggs also in lung, CNS
S. japonicum	China; Japan; Philippines	″ ″
S. haematobium	Africa; Mediterranean	Eggs in bladder → haematuria bladder cancer

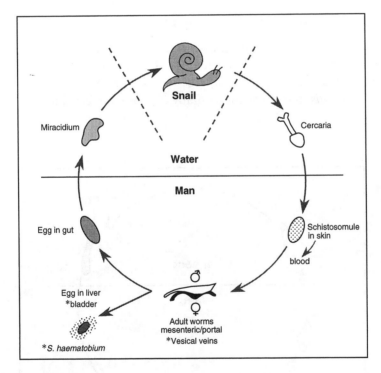

Fig. 6.1 The schistosome life cycle.

crustacean (crab). The adult worms settle mainly in the lungs, forming cysts and occasionally causing bronchopneumonia.

Nematodes

Filarial nematodes

These thread-like worms have a simple life cycle, involving a sexual stage giving birth to microfilarial larvae in the mammalian host, and an insect vector in which the larval stages develop (Fig. 6.2). The four major filarial pathogens of man differ mainly in the sites at which larvae, adult worms, and microfilaria become deposited (Table 6.4).

Other filarial nematodes causing human infection are *Mansonella Streptocerca*, *M. perstans* and *M. ozzardi* but are of little medical importance.

Non-filarial nematodes with a tissue phase

The Guinea worm *Dracunculus*, in which the larvae mature in the crustacean *Cyclops* and the adult worms live under the skin, has the dubious distinction of being the largest nematode of man, growing up to a metre or more in length. *Trichinella spiralis*, though acquired orally (by eating infected meat), causes its

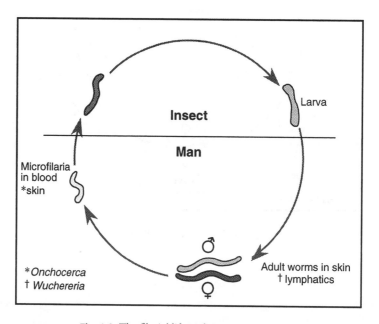

Fig. 6.2 The filarial life cycle.

Table 6.4 Major characteristics of the human filarial nematodes

Species	Vector and distribution	Disease features
Onchocerca volvulus	Simulium fly Africa; S. America	Adult worms in skin nodules Microfilariae in skin Larvae in eye → 'river blindness'
Wuchereria bancrofti Brugia malayi	Mosquito (Africa); (E. Asia)	Adult worms in lymphatics → lymphoedema → elephantiasis Microfilariae in blood
Loa loa	Mango fly (Africa)	Adult worms in eye, subcutaneous Microfilariae in blood → CNS

Table 6.5 Major characteristics of the human intestinal nematodes

Species	Site infected	Principal pathology
Ascaris lumbricoides	Small intestine, with migration to liver, heart, lungs, and back to gut	Intestinal obstruction; Allergic pneumonitis
Trichuris trichiura	Colon, caecum	Diarrhoea; rectal prolapse
Enterobius vermicularis	Caecum, rectum	Anal pruritus
Ancylostoma duodenalis (hookworm)	Small intestine, attached to mucosa	anaemia Itch;
Necator americanus	" "	" "
Strongyloides stercoralis	" "	Malabsorption May disseminate in immunodeficient individuals

main pathology when the larvae encyst in striated and (rarely) cardiac muscle. A somewhat similar process, affecting several tissues (liver, brain, eye), occurs with the dog worm *Toxocara canis*, giving rise to 'visceral larva migrans'.

Intestinal nematodes

Most species of intestinal nematodes are acquired orally or via the skin and spread by the faecal route without an intermediate host. They include the heaviest and most widespread of all helminth infections and significantly impair growth and cognitive development of infected children (see Table 6.5). For example, individuals have been found harbouring up to 1000 *Ascaris* worms which may be up to 30 cm long, the females being capable of laying 200 000

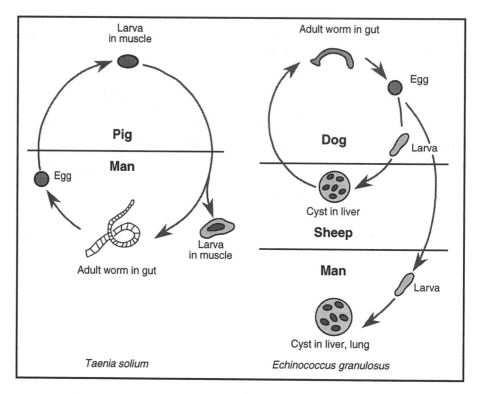

Fig. 6.3 Cestode life cycles.

eggs daily. The total annual egg output for China alone has been estimated as over 10 000 tons.

Cestodes (tapeworms)

The adults are flat, segmented worms, each segment containing both male and female organs. Their life cycle usually requires an intermediate host in which a cystic stage develops (Fig. 6.3).

Adult tapeworms in the gut, though they may reach up to 10 metres in length, usually cause only mild digestive symptoms. However, in two cases the cystic larval stages can be pathogenic when they infect vital organs.

1 *Taenia solium* (the pork tapeworm). The adult tapeworm lives in man and the normal intermediate host is the pig, which becomes infected by swallowing eggs from human faeces. However, man may also act as an intermediate host. After swallowing eggs, these release larvae in the duodenum which are carried via the blood to muscle, CNS, and eye where they form cysts with pain, fever and neurological symptoms.

2 *Echinococcus granulosus*. The adult worms are found in dogs and the larval cysts in the liver and other organs of sheep and humans. These *hydatid* cysts may contain 'daughter' cysts and several litres of fluid, and in addition to pressure effects they can induce immunopathology if they rupture (see Chapters 22 and 34). *Echinococcus multilocularis* produces rapid-growing invasive cysts; the normal animal hosts are foxes and rodents.

7 Prions

Several separate observations during more than 70 years led to the identification of a novel form of pathogen—the prion. The name, coined by Stanley Prusiner in 1982, represents the existence of a **prot**ein that is **in**fectious, and the current concept is that prions are proteins of about 50 000 kDa molecular weight, present in normal brain tissue and in an altered form in a variety of neurodegenerative diseases characterized by spongy vacuolation and amyloid plaques in grey matter (see Chapter 30). Since many of these diseases were hitherto attributed to 'slow viruses' and since it is extremely hard to eliminate the possibility of a minute amount of nucleic acid associated with the protein (the 'virion' theory), some authorities are still unconvinced, but the evidence for prions as pathogens is now fairly overwhelming. Table 7.1 shows some of the key steps in the development of the prion theory.

The really novel biological aspect of this remarkable sequence of events is the idea that protein *conformation*, for example, the proportion of α- to β-pleated sheet, rather than just amino-acid sequence, can determine function, including the initiation of fatal degenerative diseases. It focuses attention on the role of *chaperones*—the molecules that regulate the folding of proteins into their secondary and tertiary structure. Perhaps this will be the clue that leads eventually to the development of drug-based therapies.

A striking feature of the pathology of prion diseases is the apparent lack of immune responses to the damaged brain tissue. This is not because prion proteins (PrPs) are not immunogenic—indeed an antiserum to the 27–30 kDa fragment of PrP^{Sc} (the form of PrP in prion disease) was used to detect it in suspected prion diseases—but probably because, in the absence of inflammation and breaching of the blood–brain barrier, brain antigens do not make contact with lymphocytes. However, the use of a vaccine that induced immune responses in the vicinity of altered prions would clearly be a risky matter. Avoidance of the known routes of spread appears, at present, to be the only effective approach to reducing the numbers of cases.

Table 7.1 A brief history of prion biology

1920–1	Creutzfeldt and Jakob described a form of dementia (CJD) characterized by spongiform encephalopathy.
1930	CJD shown to be familial (i.e. genetic) as well as infectious.
1947	Scrapie (a similar disease of sheep) transmitted by an agent resistant to heat and formalin (which inactivate viruses).
1954	Scrapie attributed to a 'slow virus'.
1959	Kuru (a similar disease restricted to brain-eaters in New Guinea) attributed to a slow virus.
1966	Kuru transmitted to primates from diseased human brain.
1968	CJD transmitted to primates from diseased human brain.
1970	Scrapie 'agent' shown to be resistant to UV (which destroys DNA).
1978	CJD agent shown to be UV-resistant.
1982	Scrapie agent shown to be susceptible to proteolytic treatments; named 'prion' or prion protein (PrP).
1984–6	Two forms of PrP described: PrP^c (in normal cells) and PrP^{Sc} (in prion disease), differing in conformation. PrP^{Sc} is richer in β-pleated sheets and poorer in α-helices, is deposited as fibrils, and converts neighbouring PrP^c to PrP^{Sc}—a true infectious process. Antibody raised in mice to a 30 kDa fragment of PrP.
1985–6	Amyloid fibres in prion disease shown to be composed of PrP.
1986	Bovine spongiform encephalopathy (BSE) described in British cattle (spread from sheep scrapie by bone/meat feeding?).
1988	UK ban on contaminated cattle feed.
1989	Familial prion disease shown to be due to a mutation in the PrP gene.
	UK ban on 'specified offal' in beef for human consumption.
1993	Deletion of PrP gene in mice prevents induction of prion disease.
	Peak of BSE epidemic in UK.
1993–7	CJD transmitted by human growth hormone, pituitary gonadotrophin, dura mater grafts.
1995	A new form, variant CJD (vCJD), described in young humans, spread from cattle BSE.
	European Union bans British beef.
1994–7	Prion-like proteins found in fungi.
1998	Last recorded death from kuru.

8 Disease: virulence and susceptibility

The term 'infectious disease' implies the existence of not merely a parasite but a *pathogen* that makes people ill—that is, they develop symptoms, which may even be fatal. This is a sign that somewhere tissue has been damaged, either grossly in terms of structure or more subtly by a disturbance of function. This is the realm of *pathology* and the question, as hinted in Chapter 1, is therefore: why should a parasite induce pathology?

The answer is not as obvious as it might seem, and in Chapters 13 and 22 you will learn the surprising fact that in many infections it is actually the immune system that causes much of the pathology. However, in this chapter we will discuss those elements in the pathogen that predispose to disease, which are collectively known as *virulence factors*. Some of these have been mentioned in Chapter 3 in relation to bacteria, but as Table 8.1 shows, there are many others.

Genomics

Recent molecular biological advances have facilitated the precise identification of many microbial virulence factors, particularly those involving proteins. The complete sequences (DNA or RNA) of the relatively small genomes of viruses have been available for some time, but those of at least 50 bacteria and some eucaryotes, right up to man, have now been completely sequenced, making it possible to start analysing gene function, the effect of mutations, etc.—the science of *genomics* (Table 8.2). More relevant to understanding their actual function during infection is the analysis of all messenger RNAs transcribed—the *transcriptome*. And finally the protein products themselves, which may be modified post-transcriptionally, can be studied—the *proteome*. Given a full knowledge of genome, transcriptome, and proteome for a particular pathogen, which will inevitably include all protein antigens and virulence factors, extraordinary opportunities are opened up for accurate epidemiology, diagnosis, comparison of clinical and laboratory strains, evolutionary studies, and drug and vaccine design—a new era in the study of infectious disease (Table 8.3).

Virulence factors that are mainly carbohydrate or lipid cannot, of course, be directly deduced from the genome, but some of their structures are well established, for example bacterial lipopolysaccharide (see Fig. 13.1), a molecule with a number of variants that has so far eluded attempts to attack it through drugs or a vaccine.

Table 8.1 Some important virulence factors

Mechanism	Result	Example
Cytopathic organism	Destruction of host cells	Lytic viruses polio, flu; Malaria
Release of exotoxins	Various (see Table 8.4)	Staphylococci, tetanus, cholera
Infect lymphocytes and dendritic cells	Inactivate immunity	HIV, measles
Capsule	Block phagocytosis	Staph; strep; Haemophilus, Meningococcus
Adhesion factors	Prevent removal	*E. coli*; *Mycoplasma Neisseria* (pili)
Endotoxin in cell wall	Macrophage stimulation cytokine release; shock	*Salmonella* Meningococcus
Ciliary toxin	Inhibit cilia in bronchi	*B. pertussis*
Antigenic variation	Escape from immunity	Flu, HIV, *Borrelia Trypanosoma*
Plasmid exchange	Resist chemotherapy	*Staph. aureus*
Protease	Destroys IgA	*Neisseria*
Protein A	Blocks IgG	*Staphylococcus*
Urease	Protects against acid	*Helicobacter*
Elastase	Inhibits complement	*Pseudomonas*
IL-10-like molecule	Inhibits other cytokines	EBV
Reduce MHC	Avoid cytotoxic T cells	CMV
Inhibit killing mechanisms	Intracellular survival	TB, *Listeria, Brucella*
Induce granuloma	Elude immune system	TB
Induce cyst formation	″ ″ ″	*Echinococcus*

Genetics of host susceptibility

Genetic differences on the host side also contribute to the occurrence and severity of disease, though these are frequently multigenic and more difficult to investigate than when they can be accounted for by a single gene, as is sometimes the case. A hint of this will be given if the disease, or some element of it, segregates in a Mendelian fashion, as was observed in mice with suceptibility/resistance to a range of intracellular infections (BCG, *Leishmania, S. typhimurium*), which

Table 8.2 Some applications of genomics to the study of infectious diseases

Analysis	Applications	Examples
Genome (DNA) 'comparative genomics'	Discovery of genes:	
	– new families	Lipid metabolism in *M. tuberculosis*
	– unknown function	*E. coli*
	– 'core genome'	*M. tuberculosis, Brucella, Plasmodium*
	Comparison of genes:	
	– strains versus species	*M. tuberculosis*
	– pathogen versus host	Staph, Strep, *M. tuberculosis*
	Evolutionary studies:	
	– of pathogen	*Neisseria, Yersinia*
	– of host range	*Yersinia, Listeria M. tuberculosis*
	Virulence factors	Many
	Vaccination	DNA vaccines (many pathogens)
Transcriptome (mRNA) 'expression genomics'	Response to external factors:	
	– environmental stress	*Salmonella, Campylobacter*
	– site of infection	*S. pneumoniae*
	– oxygen	*M. tuberculosis*
	– host defences	*H. pylori*/acid
		M. tuberculosis/ macrophages
		Trypanosomes/antigen variation
	Drugs and drug resistance	*M. tuberculosis*, etc.
Proteome (proteins)	Protein studies:	
	– identifying new drug targets	*Plasmodium*, etc.
	– mechanisms of drug resistance	Many
	– vaccine candidates	Many
	– diagnostic tools	Many
	– immune serum	Malaria, etc.
	– T cells	*Leishmania, M. tuberculosis*, etc.

was narrowed down to a gene now known as Slc11a1 (formerly NRAMP-1), a cation-protein transporter. In the case of humans, very large studies are needed (at least 100 cases) but some single-gene links have been established (Table 8.4). An encouraging recent discovery is the extraordinary similarity between the human and mouse genomes, which should allow the effects of human genes, alone or in combination, to be modelled in the laboratory with greater confidence.

Disease directly due to the pathogen

As can be seen from Table 8.1, in two situations disease is caused directly by the pathogen:

(1) pathogens that destroy cells (*cytopathic*), predominantly viruses

(2) pathogens that release *toxins*, predominantly bacteria.

Table 8.3 Some important species whose genomes have been sequenced

Organism	Disease	Genome size (MB)
Homo sapiens		~2900
Mus musculus (mouse)		~2500
Danio rerio (zebrafish)		~1700
Schistosoma mansoni	Schistosomiasis	~270
Caenorhabditis elegans		97
Aspergillus fumigatus	Aspergillosis	~30–35
Plasmodium falciparum	Cerebral malaria	23
Entamoeba histolytica	Amoebic dysentery	~20
Trypanosoma brucei	African sleeping sickness	~35
Mycobacterium tuberculosis	Tuberculosis	4.4
Mycobacterium leprae	Leprosy	3.1
Vibrio cholerae	Cholera	4.0
Neisseria meningitidis	Meningitis	2.18
Streptococcus pyogenes	Toxic shock/rheumatic fever, necrotizing fasciitis	1.85
Helicobacter pylori	Peptic ulcer, gastric cancer	1.66
Borrelia burgdorferi	Lyme disease	1.44
Treponema pallidum	Syphilis	1.14
Mycoplasma genitalium	Urethritis	0.58
Hepadnaviridae	E.g. hepatitis B	0.003
Poxviridae	E.g. smallpox	~0.2
Filoviridae	E.g. Ebola	0.012 (RNA)
Retroviridae	E.g. HIV	0.003–0.009 (RNA)

Cytopathic infections

In Chapter 2 (see especially Fig. 2.4) we described how some viruses spread by killing the host cell. Sometimes the damage is mainly in the cytoplasm, with inhibition of essential nucleic acid or protein synthesis, sometimes mainly in the cell membrane, resulting in lysis. Sometimes the cell is merely 'rounded up', separated from its neighbours and washed away, leaving a very sore mucous membrane; this is what happens to the nose and throat with the common cold viruses. Pathologists recognize the signs of cell damage as *cloudy swelling*, the presence

Table 8.4 Some human disease susceptibility/resistance genes

Genes	Disease association
HbS (sickle cell)	*P. falciparum* malaria
Duffy blood group negativity	*P. vivax* malaria
CCR5, CCR2 (chemokine receptors)	HIV/AIDS
Interferon γ receptor; IL-12	Disseminated BCG; *Salmonella*, Atypical mycobacteria
MBL-2, FcγRII	Acute bacterial infection
HLA-DR	TB, leprosy, Hepatitis B, Malaria
CSF, IL-4, IL-5, IL-9, IL-13 region	Egg output in schistosomiasis
Vitamin D receptor, *SLC11A1*	TB

of *inclusion bodies*, or the formation of multi-cellular *giant cells* and *syncytia*. It was also mentioned in Chapter 2 that some viruses can *transform* cells into a tumour, which should clearly be included as a form of pathology, though on a much slower time-scale.

Cytopathic effects are not restricted to viruses, they are seen also in infection with other intracellular organisms such as *Chlamydia*, *Rickettsia*, *Mycoplasma* and, over a longer period of time, mycobacteria—though in the last case the cell involved (the macrophage) is readily replaceable and this is not the main cause of the pathology, most of which is immunological. The malaria parasite is unusual in growing inside and destroying firstly liver cells and subsequently red cells; the damage to the liver is insignificant but the destruction of red cells can lead to severe anaemia. Hookworms feeding on blood from the intestinal epithelium can also cause a remarkable degree of anaemia.

Most extracellular parasites are too small to cause trouble by their simple presence, but some of the worms are large enough to obstruct vital organs. Examples are the roundworms *Ascaris* (intestine, bile duct) and *Wuchereria* (lymphatics), while the 'hydatid' cysts formed by the tapeworm *Echinococcus* can cause mechanical problems in the liver and lung.

Toxins

Several of the most acute and dangerous bacterial diseases are caused not by the bacteria themselves but by the toxins they secrete. Secreted toxins are known as *exotoxins*, as distinct from the *endotoxins* that are an integral part of the cell wall (see LPS, Fig. 3.2); the way endotoxins cause pathology will be discussed later (see Chapter 13).

Bacterial exotoxins are interesting for a number of reasons. They include some of the most toxic molecules in existence; for example one milligram of botulinum toxin (beloved of detective story writers) is calculated to be enough to kill a million guinea-pigs. Vaccines against the exotoxin of tetanus and diphtheria are among the most successful vaccines available, and must have saved hundreds of millions of lives from these rapidly fatal diseases. Toxins are often coded for by extra-chromosomal DNA, sometimes in the form of plasmids, sometimes of bacterial viruses (phages). Because of their well-studied mode of action, several toxins have become valuable laboratory reagents, one—botulinum (Botox)— having even found its way into the beauty industry. Finally, there is the question, why should bacteria secrete molecules, some of which are almost guaranteed to kill their host?

To take the last point first, some exotoxins undoubtedly help the bacteria to spread through the tissues or to get out of the body (Table 8.5). For bacteria that are not normally parasitic (e.g. tetanus) one could argue that death of the host is irrelevant. The impression remains that some toxin-secreting bacteria are 'over-doing it' a bit, and it will be interesting to see how those bacteria fare whose toxins have been genetically engineered away, as is now being done in molecular biology laboratories—for example with the deletion of the α toxin from *Clostridium perfringens*, which considerably reduces its virulence.

The modes of action of exotoxins are very diverse, but can be classified under five main headings. Table 8.6 illustrates these, bringing out the fact that some toxins consist of more than one subunit, usually one to bind (B) to a cell-surface receptor and one to act (A) inside the cell. Advantage has been taken of this recently, in that by replacing the binding subunit by some other molecule with very precise cell specificity (monoclonal antibodies are generally used), the toxic subunit can be directed to a particular cell such as a cancer cell—the 'magic bullet' therapy. Possibly in the future the same approach might be used to attack recalcitrant pathogens.

Table 8.5 Some exotoxins are of potential benefit to the organisms that secrete them

Organism	Toxin	Benefit to organism
Streptococcus	Streptokinase	Spread through tissues
	Hyaluronidase	Spread through tissues
	Streptolysin	Destroys phagocytes
Staphylococcus	Leucocidin	Destroys phagocytes
	Enterotoxin	Diarrhoea → spread
Bordetella pertussis	Toxin	Blocks bronchial cilia
Clostridium perfringens	Phospholipase (α toxin)	Spread through tissues
Shigella Cholera, *E. coli*	Enterotoxins	Diarrhoea → spread
Entamoeba histolytica	Toxin	Penetrates gut wall

Another way for bacterial toxins and enzymes (e.g. from *Salmonella*, *Shigella*, *Yersinia*) to gain entry to cells is by the formation of tubular structures in the membrane—a Type III ('syringe and needle') secretion mechanism by which as many as 20 different proteins can be injected at once into host cells. Many bacteria carry not only toxins and secretion systems but also other virulence factors together in their genome or on plasmids; these *pathogenicity islands* constitute the main difference between virulent and non-virulent strains.

A few non-bacterial organisms also produce exotoxins. In one case, the protozoan *Entamoeba histolytica*, the toxin may assist the parasite to penetrate the intestinal wall and form its characteristic 'amoebic' abscesses. In another example, the fungus *Aspergillus flavus*, the toxin (aflatoxin) may contaminate food sources such as grain and nuts, and has been incriminated in the development of liver damage and liver cancer. Note that some secreted toxins (e.g. TSST-1 from *Staphylococcus aureus*) act indirectly by over-stimulating the production of cytokines by the host—that is, behaving like endotoxins (see Chapter 13).

Diarrhoea and vomiting

These common complications of intestinal infection with toxin-producing organisms are worth separate comment. Symptoms following within hours of a

Table 8.6 Bacterial exotoxins produce their effects in a variety of ways

Mode of action	Example
Lysis of cell membranes	
(1) by enzyme action	*Clostridium perfringens* (phospholipase C)
(2) by pore formation	*Staphylococcus aureus* (α toxin)
Lysis of connective tissue and fibrin	*Streptococcus pyogenes* (streptokinase, hyaluronidase)
Inhibition of protein synthesis	*Corynebacterium diphtheriae* (diphtheria toxin, B unit binds, A unit blocks ribosome function)
Raise cAMP levels leading to fluid loss	*Vibrio cholerae* (cholera toxin, B unit binds, A units raise cAMP) *E. coli*, Shigella similar *Anthrax* (also kills macrophages)
Blocking of nerve–muscle transmission	
(1) by blocking acetylcholine release	*Clostridium botulinum* ($\rightarrow$ flaccid paralysis)
(2) by overstimulation	*Clostridium tetani* ($\rightarrow$ spastic paralysis)

Table 8.7 Vomiting and diarrhoea can be due to a wide variety of infectious organisms. Often the time between exposure and symptoms is a guide to the likely cause

Organism	Common sources	Time of onset
Food poisoning (toxin in food)		
Staphylococcus aureus	Cream, meat	1–6 hrs
Bacillus cereus	Reheated food	1–20 hrs
Clostridium perfringens	Reheated meat	8–20 hrs
Clostridium botulinum	Tinned food	12–36 hrs
Infectious gastroenteritis (organisms in food)		
Rotaviruses	Faecal–oral	2–5 days
Enteroviruses	Faecal–oral	2–5 days
Shigella	Faecal–oral	1–4 days
V. cholerae	Faecal–oral	1–2 days
E. coli	Faecal–oral	1–4 days
Salmonella	Eggs, meat	1–2 days
Campylobacter	Eggs, meat	1–2 days
Yersinia	Animals	Gradual
Giardia lamblia	Faecal–oral	1–2 weeks
Entamoeba	Faecal–oral	Gradual
Cryptosporidia	Animals	Gradual

meal ('food poisoning') are usually due to toxins already present in the food, whereas if the food is merely contaminated with organisms, symptoms take a few days to appear (Table 8.7). In both cases, the symptoms can be viewed as a logical attempt on the part of the host to get rid of the cause, but they can also be life threatening, the death from dehydration that can occur within 24 hours of the onset of cholera being an extreme example. From the bacterial point of view, of course, this is an excellent method of spread. Note, however, that not all diarrhoea is caused by bacteria; it may be due to viruses, protozoa, drugs, poisons, non-infectious disease of the bowel, and even nervousness.

Tutorial **1**

At this point you should have a sufficient understanding of the major pathogens and their direct effects on their host to attempt an essay on each of the topics below. Make a list of the headings you would base your essay on and a suitable order to present them in, and compare your version with the specimen lists below.

1. Comment on this (fictional) press release.

   The malaria virus threatens to make a come-back in Northern Europe, a Junior Health Minister warned yesterday on his return from Nairobi, advising his audience to have their vaccine boost and avoid uncooked meat when abroad.

2. We would be better off without bacteria. Discuss.
3. Viruses are not really living organisms—or are they?
4. No parasite needs to make its host ill. Discuss.
5. The evolution of higher animals has not significantly affected the world of microorganisms. Discuss.

Some hints and pointers (remember, there is never one single perfect answer to an essay question).

1. The minister was incorrect in that (1) malaria is caused by a protozoan, not a virus, (2) it is not spread by uncooked meat but by a mosquito, and (3) vaccines against it are still experimental. He was correct in that (1) it was once widespread in Europe and could be again if the mosquitoes could breed there, and (2) it is definitely unwise to eat uncooked meat abroad, mainly because of contamination with bacteria and worms. (As a matter of additional interest there is no malaria in Nairobi because of its height above sea level.) Descriptions of infectious organisms in the newspapers are often full of errors.

2. Do not assume the question means only *parasitic* bacteria! It would be wise to include a discussion of the vital importance of bacteria in the evolution of life on earth, in the maintenance of ecosystems, of carbon, nitrogen, sulphur cycles, etc., and in modern molecular biology. You could mention that some antibiotics come from bacteria (though of course they might not be needed if there were no bacterial diseases!). Then you could consider the role of bacteria in ruminants, in which they are responsible for digesting cellulose (a cow's

rumen contains over 100 litres, with 10^{10} or more bacteria per millilitre). This would lead on to the human gut flora, generally considered to have a useful, though not vital, function. Finally the comparatively few bacteria that cause human disease could be discussed; it would be reasonably safe to conclude that, as individuals, we would be better off without these, though the increased lifespan that has already resulted from reducing infectious disease is causing medical and social problems at the population level.

3. A tricky question and really a matter of definition. What is life? If the ability to infect and self-replicate is sufficient, they are certainly living. But if metabolic activity is also a requirement, they are not, since they depend on their host cell to supply this. A safe compromise would be to regard them as mobile sets of genes with their own reproductive capacity—though this gets very close to including bacterial plasmids in the definition. In fact, this is an academic rather than a seriously important question.

4. Again, the short answer is that the best parasites do not make their hosts ill, and certainly do not kill them in large numbers. This might lead on to the argument that host–parasite pairs, given time, will evolve towards the most mutually beneficial relationship, the lethal parasites being only recently, or accidentally, acquired. But is this true? Some bacterial toxins may have to destroy tissues to allow the bacteria to spread. An organism may have to cause diarrhoea to get back into the water supply. Does the occasional host death matter to such organisms? Later in the book you will see that the role of the immune system has to be taken into account too, but even at this stage you could build up an interesting debate. Keeping the examiner *interested* is half the battle—you can lose far more marks by being boring (or illegible) than by the odd error of fact.

5. This is a good example of a question to which nobody knows the complete answer, since we can never know what would have happened if higher animals had not evolved. Nevertheless, there is a lot to say. You might perhaps divide your higher animals into *man* and the rest. Clearly man, with his vaccines and antibiotics, has made a huge impact—the elimination of smallpox being a really major triumph. When you know more about antibiotics, however, you will see that they are a two-edged weapon, with the ability to drive microbial evolution faster (penicillin resistance, etc.). Then there is the amazing power of genetic engineering to create mutant or recombinant microbes that never existed before, whose possibilities make yesterday's science fiction today's fact. But leaving man aside, higher animals have been useful to microbes rather than the opposite; think of the difficulty the malaria parasite would have in spreading from person to person without the help of mosquitoes (or, as some parasitologists would put it, in spreading from mosquito to mosquito without help from humans). The expansion of higher species must have opened up possibilities for the development of new viruses, since many of these are quite species specific.

Part 2

The immune system

9 External defences: entry and exit

We turn now to a consideration of the host and how it can defend itself against disease induced by pathogens. The problem is very analogous to that faced by a country at war, namely how to avoid damage by enemy agents, and in fact the solutions arrived at by nature and by governments are remarkably similar. Nature's method operates at three levels:

(1) keep pathogens out by setting up effective *external defences*;

(2) if they get in, catch and dispose of them rapidly, using an always ready and available army of cells and molecules—the *innate immune system*;

(3) if they elude capture, devote a specialized set of cells to each pathogen, able to identify it, mark it for disposal, and retain memory of the details for the future—the *adaptive immune system*.

Innate and adaptive immunity will be described in Chapters 10–25; here we shall concentrate on level 1, the external defences. To appreciate these we need first to appreciate the ways in which a pathogen might get into the body, which obviously dictate the kind of external defences required.

External defences: physical and chemical

The healthy body is surrounded by an intact layer of skin (outside) and mucous membranes (lining the hollow viscera). These are a very effective barrier against invasion by most pathogens, although some are able to get through. The secretions of the various skin glands contain quite powerful antimicrobial proteins, such as lysozyme, lactoferrin, defensins, and peroxidases. These may be produced by epithelial cells themselves, by specialized glands, or by phagocytic cells such as neutrophils and macrophages that have migrated to the site. Their action may be directly antimicrobial by enzymatic digestion of the pathogen (e.g. phospholipases) or by forming pores in the membrane (e.g. antibiotic peptides). Many of these substances are present constitutively in normal tissues, but their concentration can be greatly increased following challenge with a pathogen. Each has a broad but not unlimited antimicrobial spectrum, with activity mainly focused on bacteria, fungi, or some viruses. Simultaneous production of several different substances therefore provides coverage against a wide range of pathogens. These components of the defence system are particularly suited for dealing with the small numbers of invading organisms encountered during every-day life. Larger numbers of pathogens that overwhelm this local killing capacity have to be dealt with by other elements of the innate and adaptive immune systems, as described in later chapters.

The skin

If the continuity of the skin is lost, entry into the tissues by organisms normally resident on the surface can occur; a painful example is the common development of staphylococcal infections following a wound or burn. Alternatively, if the pathogen manages to infect a biting animal, insect, etc., entry is obviously facilitated, sometimes (e.g. a mosquito bite) directly into the bloodstream; see Table 9.1.

Unlike the skin, the linings of the respiratory, intestinal, and urogenital tracts are delicate membranes, designed to allow the exchange of substances across them. They are therefore rather more vulnerable to penetration by parasites, and

Table 9.1 Though the skin is generally an efficient barrier to pathogens, several of them do enter by this route, some of which (*) can also enter via the respiratory tract

Intact skin		
Direct attachment		Pox viruses
		Papova (wart) virus
		Dermatophytes (fungi)
	from water	Hookworm
		Leptospira
		Schistosoma
Insect bite		Yellow fever
		Typhus
		Borrelia (Lyme disease)
		*Plague
		Malaria
		Trypanosomes (African; S. American)
		Leishmania
		Roundworms (e.g. *Onchocerca*)
Animal bite		Rabies
Abrasions, wounds, burns		Staphylococci
		Streptococci
		Clostridium
		tetani (tetanus)
		perfringens (gas gangrene)
		*Anthrax

require special mechanisms to prevent this which have to be considered separately.

The respiratory tract

The inhalation of viruses, bacteria, and fungi is unavoidable. It is estimated that a normal person inhales at least 10 000 microbes daily, and a wide range of infections are acquired by this route (Table 9.2). However, it is a remarkable fact that in healthy life the terminal parts of the respiratory tract—the alveoli, where gases are exchanged—are sterile. This is achieved by a combination of mucus secretion in the lower bronchial tree and the upwardly beating action of cilia, which constantly waft this mucus up towards the pharynx, to be coughed out or swallowed; this has been vividly termed the *muco-ciliary escalator*. Its importance is illustrated by the serious lung infections suffered by patients with *cystic fibrosis*, a genetic disorder in which the mucus is too viscid to be cleared properly, resulting in distended and chronically infected airways, a condition known as bronchiectasis. Some microbes can defeat the 'escalator' either by forming firm attachments to the bronchial membranes (viruses and some bacteria) or by inhibiting the action of the cilia (mainly bacteria); see Table 9.3. Needless to say, these are among the most successful parasites of the respiratory system, responsible for many serious chest infections.

Table 9.2 Numerous infectious organisms enter the body via the respiratory route. Most cause respiratory disease, but some (*) may spread to other organs

Viruses	Adenovirus, rhinovirus, influenza, measles, mumps, rubella, VZV (chickenpox), parvovirus
Bacteria	*Staphylococci, *Streptococci, diphtheria, anthrax, *mycobacteria (TB, leprosy), *Neisseria meningitidis*, *Haemophilus influenzae*, Bordetella pertussis* (whooping cough), *mycoplasma
Fungi	*Aspergillus*, *Histoplasma*, *Blastomyces*, *Cryptococcus*

Table 9.3 Several viruses and bacteria can avoid the normal flushing actions of the muco-ciliary escalator

	Viruses	Bacteria
Attachment to respiratory epithelium	Rhinovirus Adenovirus Influenza	*Neisseria meningitidis* *Haemophilus* *Streptococcus pneumoniae* Mycoplasma
Inactivation of ciliary function	Influenza Measles	*Haemophilus* *Bordetella pertussis* Mycoplasma

The alveolar spaces also contain the hydrophilic surfactant proteins SP-A and SP-D which can recognize the surface carbohydrates of pathogens, leading to aggregation and enhanced uptake by phagocytes. Between the mucous layer and the epithelium lies a thin layer of liquid containing many of the antimicrobial proteins mentioned above, notably lysozyme, lactoferrin, and secretory leukoproteinase inhibitor (SLPI), which act synergistically, and also numerous low molecular weight antimicrobial peptides including defensins, cathelicidin, and various neutrophil-derived peptides. There is some evidence that the level of these antimicrobial molecules may differ from person to person, which may partly explain the very different individual susceptibilities to respiratory infection. The fact that many of these peptides are inhibited at high salt concentrations, such as are found in the lung in cystic fibrosis, may be a further contributory cause of the repeated respiratory infections in this condition. A further point of interest is that some of these peptides may become available for therapeutic purposes.

The highly important part played by the immune system in such infections is described in later chapters, but it is worth mentioning here that respiratory infections are one of the most common consequences of *immunodeficiency*.

The intestine

Like the air we breathe, food and water are inevitably contaminated with microbes, though proper cooking and water filtering can reduce this contamination substantially. The first difficulty encountered by microbes on their way to the intestine is the very strong acidity of the stomach contents—about pH 2. The value of this in killing bacteria is illustrated by the fact that swallowing a teaspoonful of sodium bicarbonate is enough to lower the minimum infective dose of cholera or salmonella organisms by a factor of 10 000. The other main mechanisms for ridding the intestinal tract of microbes are vomiting and diarrhoea—though it must be said that these are (a) unpleasant and potentially dangerous to the host and (b) useful to the pathogen in assisting transmission by what is aptly referred to as the 'faecal–oral' route (Table 9.4). To the surprise of many physicians, it has recently become apparent that one bacterium, *Helicobacter pylori*, adapted to life in the stomach by the production of urease, may be the cause of about 80% of gastric and duodenal ulcers. The detergent action of the bile salts is also thought to destroy many bacteria, and there are specialized protective antibodies in the gut which will be described in Chapter 16. As in the respiratory tract, antimicrobial peptides, lysozyme, phospholipases, etc. can be found in the gut, secreted in response to bacteria by the Paneth cells. The possibility that the 'normal' gut flora prevent overgrowth by more virulent bacteria has already been mentioned (see Chapter 3).

Table 9.4 The faecal–oral route is a major pathway of spread for intestinal pathogens, both human–human and animal–human

Faecal–oral route	Other routes
Enteroviruses	Milk
Polio, Coxsackie, Echo, hepatitis A	*Listeria*
Rotavirus	*Brucella*
E. coli	Tuberculosis (*M. bovis*)
	Pets
Salmonella	Cats
Shigella	*Toxoplasma*
Cholera	Dogs
Amoeba	*Toxocara*
Giardia	Hydatid worm
	Meat and other foods
	Taenia (tapeworm)
	Trichinella
	Ascaris

The urogenital tract

Normally the urine is sterile, and any organisms that make their way in through the urethra are flushed out again. However, because of the shortness of the urethra in females, episodes of bacterial infection in the bladder (cystitis) are fairly common, and the same is true when proper voiding of urine is impeded. Ascending infection is limited by the production in the kidney of an antibacterial peptide β defensin-1, present in normal urine (10–100 ug/ml) and increased in response to infection. Similar peptides are produced in the vagina, cervix, and uterus; their concentration fluctuates during the menstrual cycle, suggesting a regulatory role for hormones. One type of bacterium, the gonococcus, possesses specialized structures (pili) that allow it to cling to the urethral wall, which explains why it is mainly sexually transmitted.

The eye

Shortly after the First World War, Alexander Fleming noticed that human tears, saliva, and plasma contained something that destroyed the walls of certain bacteria. He had discovered *lysozyme*, an enzyme that cleaves the peptidoglycan of Gram-positive bacteria (see Fig. 3.2) and also the chitin of fungi. Together with the flushing action of the tears, it helps to keep the surface of the eye free of infection, though many bacteria are resistant to it and some of them, particularly the chlamydiae, can persist indefinitely in the cells of the conjunctiva. It is

Table 9.5 The principal routes of spread by pathogens; note the risk of transferring infections by blood transfusion

Contact	Most skin infections
	Epstein–Barr virus (saliva)
Coughing, sneezing	Most respiratory infections
Faecal, diarrhoea	Most intestinal infections
Sexual	Herpesvirus (HSV 2)
	HIV
	Neisseria gonorrhoeae
	Treponema pallidum (syphilis)
	Trachoma
Blood and blood products	Hepatitis B, C
	HIV
	Malaria
Insect or animal bites	(see Table 9.1)

Table 9.6 The major arthropod vector-borne infections

Disease	Vector
Viruses	
Dengue	Mosquito
Yellow fever	Mosquito
Tick-borne encephalitis	Tick
Rickettsiae	
Typhus	Flea, louse
Spotted fevers	Tick
Bacteria	
Plague	Flea
Relapsing fever	Louse
Lyme disease	Tick
Protozoa	
Malaria	Mosquito
Leishmaniasis	Sandfly
Sleeping sickness	Tsetse fly
Chagas' disease	Reduviid bug
Helminths	
Onchocerciasis	Simulium fly
Filariasis	Mosquito
Loasis	Mango fly

interesting that it was also Fleming who later discovered the first fungal molecule that can attack the bacterial cell wall—penicillin.

How pathogens exit

A pathogen that cannot survive free in the environment—a virus, for instance—can only get into its host by getting out of another host. Thus for many pathogens it is vital to find a means of exit. Table 9.5 lists the main escape routes used by pathogens, with some typical examples of each. You will note that the type of spread influences the pattern of disease considerably. Thus an upper respiratory virus that spreads by aerosol (e.g. sneezes) can only maintain its presence where the host population is reasonably dense. Towns are ideal for this, and crowded train carriages are particularly efficient. In very thinly populated or isolated areas, spread by an insect vector is a practical solution (mosquitoes can fly up to 50 miles). Urogenital transmission obviously calls for very intimate contact. Perhaps the most unusual form of spread is the eating of the brains of dead ancestors, which transmits the prions that are thought to cause the degenerative central nervous disease *kuru*, an early example of spongiform encephalopthy in humans (see Chapter 7 for the link with BSE and vCJD).

A note on vectors

Vectors, particularly blood-feeding arthropods, have been mentioned in relation to both the entry and exit of pathogens. Their importance can be judged from Table 9.6. Note the slight overlap between *vectors*, which simply transmit pathogens from one host to another, and *intermediate hosts*, in which larval stages develop; strictly speaking, man is the intermediate host of malaria, mosquito the definitive one!

10 The immune system: introduction

In Chapter 9 it was emphasized that defence against pathogens operates at several levels, both before and after they get into the body. The remainder of this book will be concerned with those that do get in, and it is here that the *immune system* comes into play. This is the name given to a complex network of organs, cells, and molecules scattered throughout the body, whose function is dealing with invading infectious organisms. To work properly, it requires three sets of components:

(1) a *recognition* system to identify the presence of the invader; this is carried out at the molecular level by various recognition molecules;

(2) a *disposal* system to kill or otherwise eliminate the threat from the invader; disposal is carried out at both molecular and cellular levels;

(3) a *communication* system to coordinate the activities of the various recognition and disposal elements.

As was pointed out earlier, this is very much the way a country defends itself against enemy agents: (1) trained observers identify them, (2) weapons knock them out, and (3) radio keeps everyone in touch. And in a very similar way to an army, all these immune components are characterized by a high degree of *mobility*, which makes sense, considering that it is impossible to know in advance where the invader will choose to attack—a feature unique to the immune system.

Recognition molecules

Pursuing the analogy with the armed forces, one can imagine that an invader could be recognized simply because it 'looks unusual', or because it is clearly 'foreign', or because it corresponds to a precise 'known face' in some central filing system. At the same time, care must be taken not to mis-recognize and dispose of members of our own side. In immunological jargon, 'our own side' is referred to as *self* (e.g. self molecules, self cells, etc.), and everything else as *non-self*. Recognition is thus essentially a problem of distinguishing self from non-self. Unfortunately no single recognition unit can achieve this, nor is there any way of infallibly distinguishing harmful from harmless microorganisms. Recognition molecules that recognize a variety of foreign invaders are sometimes referred to as *non-specific* (although *less* specific would be a more accurate term), while those that can unerringly pick out one individual from thousands of others are called *specific*—both these terms being relative.

In later chapters you will see that non-specific recognition is characteristic of the *innate* immune system, exemplified by the phagocytic cells, while specific recognition is typical of the *adaptive* immune system, based on the lymphocyte. You will also see that the distinction of self from non-self is a more serious problem for the adaptive system, because of its millions of different recognition molecules, which are individually able to recognize virtually any type or shape of molecule, harmless or otherwise, whereas those of the phagocytes seem to be particularly responsive to microbial molecules that spell danger (see Chapters 11 and 12 for more on this).

Not all the recognition molecules are equally well understood. Those of the adaptive immune system have been very thoroughly studied; they are proteins and a great deal is known about their genes, sequences, three-dimensional shapes, etc. The recognition molecules of the innate immune system have only been identified recently and the list is probably still incomplete. Much more will be said about these molecules in later chapters. Meanwhile Table 10.1

Table 10.1 The principal recognition molecules of the immune system. Note that some of them act together, e.g. antibody and complement, the T cell receptor and MHC molecules

Molecule and location	Nature	Structures recognized
Receptors on phagocytic cells	Mostly protein	General microbial features, e.g. bacterial sugars Most foreign or denatured molecules, e.g. carbon, effete red cells Microbial DNA, RNA
Receptors on natural killer cells	Protein	Virus-infected cells and some tumour cells
Complement	Numerous proteins	(1) Some bacterial cell walls (2) Antibody bound to antigen
Major histocompatibility complex (MHC) molecules	Protein	Short intracellular peptides (transported to cell surface and presented to T cell)
T cell receptor (on T cells)	Protein	Short peptides bound to MHC Glycolipids bound to CD1
Antibody (on B cells)	Protein (immunoglobulin)	Three-dimensional shape of proteins, carbohydrates, etc.

summarizes their main features. You will see that between them they are able to recognize virtually every component of any conceivable pathogen.

Disposal mechanisms

The need to dispose of foreign material goes back to the earliest forms of cellular life. For example, an amoeba swimming in the sea needs to eat, and eating involves (1) recognition of what is food and (2) some process for getting it inside the amoeba ('endocytosis'). As animals increased in complexity, developing internal cavities and a blood circulation, not every cell needed to take in food particles in this way; instead a population of specialized cells has been retained, with properties remarkably like the primitive amoeba. In vertebrates these are the *phagocytes* (or 'eating cells')—perhaps the single most important component of our defence system. As Table 10.1 indicates, phagocytic cells have their own recognition molecules built into their surface, but also take advantage of more recently evolved recognition molecules that circulate in the blood, such as complement and antibody (see Chapters 11 and 16).

Phagocytic cells are particularly effective in disposing of bacterial and fungal infection, less so with protozoa, and of course far too small to take in worms. They are also relatively ineffective against viruses, which spend so much of their time inside the cells of the host. Two further developments go some way to filling this gap. Some phagocytes, and also some non-phagocytic cells, are able to attach to their target and kill it from the outside; this is often referred to as *extracellular killing*, and when the attachment is mediated by antibody, as *antibody-dependent cellular cytotoxicity* (ADCC). The latter may operate against worms, but this is still controversial. In the case of virus-infected cells, extracellular killing is carried out by two specialized types of cell—the natural killer (NK) cell and the cytotoxic T lymphocyte, often known as the CTL. How these cells detect the presence of viruses inside a host cell and how they then kill both cell and virus is described in Chapters 17 and 19.

When the object to be disposed of is a molecule rather than a whole microbe, for example a bacterial toxin, it is often sufficient merely to *neutralize* it. Antibody is the best-studied neutralizing molecule, but there are others (Table 10.2).

Communication: cell contact and cytokines

Few cells in the immune system act entirely on their own; much of what they do is under the influence of signals from other cells—to divide, to stop dividing, to migrate, to differentiate into effector cells, to secrete antibody, etc. These signals are delivered in two distinct ways: (1) by the interaction of cell-surface molecules brought together by cell–cell contact, and (2) by soluble molecules that can act at

Table 10.2 The principal disposal mechanisms

Disposal mechanism	Effective against
Phagocytosis, *intracellular killing	Extracellular bacteria, extracellular fungi, some protozoa
Extracellular killing	
(1) Natural killer cells	Intracellular viruses
(2) Cytotoxic T cells	〃 〃 and bacteria
(3) Antibody-dependent	
by granulocytes	Worms
by natural killer cells	Intracellular viruses (?)
	Other infections (?)
Neutralization	
by antibody	Exotoxins, viruses
Lysis	
by complement	Some bacteria, viruses, protozoa
by high-density lipoprotein	Some trypanosomes

* Note that phagocytosis is not always followed by killing, since some bacteria, fungi, and protozoa have specialized mechanisms for avoiding this; see Chapter 13.

a distance—in which case the immune system functions rather like the endocrine system, with its set of hormones to regulate the activities of other cells. In the case of the immune system, these hormone-like molecules are called *cytokines* (Fig. 10.1), a term that covers a growing list of molecules with a bewildering array of overlapping functions. Table 10.3 summarizes what they have in common, and a list of the main cytokines of relevance to infectious disease can be found in the following chapter (Table 11.2).

For historical reasons, cytokine nomenclature is not very logical; thus the *interferons* were named because they interfere with virus replication, *tumour necrosis factor* because it causes (some) tumours in mice to shrivel up, the *colony-stimulating factors* because they affect the growth of bone marrow cells in culture, *chemokines* because they induce cell movement (chemotaxis) towards them; however, all these molecules have several other important activities as well. Most new cytokines added to the list are nowadays called by the more non-committal name *interleukin* (i.e. 'between white cells') plus a number, and if they were to be discovered now, probably they would all be called interleukins.

Their effects are so widespread that cytokines will be mentioned in practically every chapter from now on. However, one rather unexpected finding is worth mentioning here, which is that there seems to be a link between these molecules and certain parasites. For example, some bacteria, protozoa, and worms appear to respond to cytokines, generally by increased growth. Even stranger is the fact that some viruses contain genes for cytokines or cytokine receptors, which they use to send confusing signals to the immune system. Immunologists are only

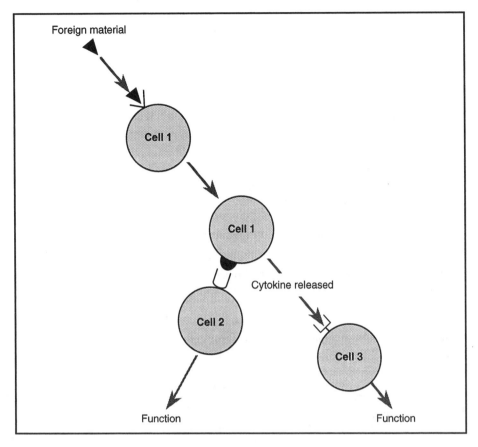

Fig. 10.1 The cells of the immune system are in permanent communication with each other, either by contact or through a network of small molecules called cytokines. In the example shown here, cell 1 has recognized foreign material and is sending signals to cell 3 to dispose of it. Meanwhile cells 1 and 2 are communicating via surface-bound molecules.

half-joking when they complain that parasites know more about immunology than they do!

Communication by cell–cell contact is of course something the endocrine system *cannot* carry out, since its cells are fixed in the endocrine organs. Indeed the immune system is the only one whose cells are constantly on the move. You will read much more about cell interactions when we consider the T and B lymphocytes in Chapters 17 and 19.

Innate and adaptive immunity

As mentioned in Chapter 9, the immune system divides conveniently into two parts—the *innate* and the *adaptive* immune systems—which differ in a number

Table 10.3 Cytokines, the communication molecules of the immune system, have several properties in common. Note that they somewhat resemble hormones, but not in all respects (see points 2, 5, 7)

1. They are proteins or glycoproteins, with molecular weights generally in the 10–30 kDa range.
2. Each of them can be produced by more than one type of cell, but usually in response to a stimulus.
3. They do not specifically recognize particular microbial molecules; thus their effects are non-specific with respect to the pathogen.
4. They bind to cell-surface receptors on the 'target' cell, which send signals to the nucleus and induce various functions.
5. Each cytokine has effects, often different, on several target cell types; however, two cytokines can sometimes have identical effects.
6. They often enhance each other's effects (synergy) or oppose each other.
7. There are soluble inhibitors (often free receptors) to restrict their effects to the immediate microenvironment of the producing cell.

Table 10.4 The division of the immune system into innate and adaptive components is based on several important differences

	Innate immunity	Adaptive immunity
Evolutionary origin	Earliest animals all invertebrates and vertebrates	Vertebrates only
Principal cells	Phagocytes	Lymphocytes
Principal molecules	Complement Cytokines	Antibody Cytokines
Specificity of recognition	Broad	*Very high
Speed of action	Rapid (minutes, hours)	Slow (days)
Development of memory	No	*Yes

* High specificity and memory are the hallmarks of adaptive immunity.

of important ways. A comparison (Table 10.4) shows that with innate immunity the emphasis is on disposal, while recognition is comparatively 'across the board' in its specificity. On the other hand adaptive immunity, which evolved much more recently, features an extremely high degree of specificity of recognition, different for individual cells, while adding relatively less in the way of new disposal mechanisms, often leaving this task to the innate system. In the following chapters, these two types of immunity will be described in considerable detail, but it should be borne in mind that in vertebrates, which possess both, the two systems are integrated, interacting with each other at many levels and employing both cell–cell contact and cytokines to do so. A further complication is that between the two extremes of the innate . . . adaptive spectrum (e.g. macrophages . . . T cells) are a number of cells with intermediate properties, inhabiting a sort of 'grey area' in terminology. The best example of this is the natural killer (NK) cell, to be described in Chapter 11, but there are others, including some sub-populations of T lymphocytes that do not carry the 'normal' T cell receptor molecules.

Another important difference between innate and adaptive immune processes has to do with the *time* factor. In a nutshell, innate immunity acts rapidly, while adaptive immune responses, because they involve an element of cell proliferation, tend to be slower off the mark. For example, the activation of complement and phagocytosis by macrophages (innate) occurs within minutes, while the production of antibody (adaptive), which requires two different kinds of lymphocyte and several cycles of cell division, can take a week or more. Fortunately lymphocyte responses display *memory*, ensuring that a subsequent response to the same pathogen occurs much faster. Thus the adaptive immune response is more flexible and vigorous, so much so that it requires quite sophisticated *regulatory* mechanisms to stop it going on too long or causing damage to its possessor—also a possibility with some innate immune mechanisms (see Chapters 13 and 20). We shall discuss the workings of adaptive immunity in detail in Chapters 15–19.

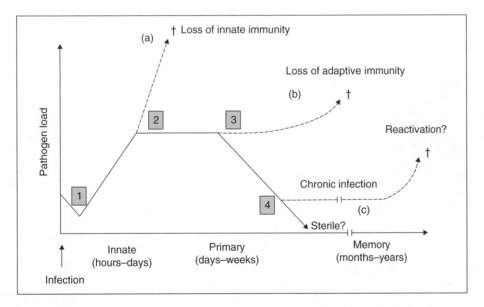

Fig. 10.2 Time course of typical infections in (a) mice lacking polymorphs and mobile macrophages, (b) mice lacking T and B lymphocytes, (c) normal mice, illustrating that natural immunity is required for early control and adaptive immunity for eventual recovery. † denotes death of host.

Since higher animals possess both innate and adaptive immune systems, it was always assumed, very reasonably, that both systems are important for optimal resistance to infection. Nowadays this question can be studied directly by using animals (usually mice) deficient in one or other system, or both. Observations can also be made on humans lacking various immune components. The effect of such deficiencies varies considerably from infection to infection, but a generalized picture might look something like Fig. 10.2, which shows the growth of an imaginary pathogen in three kinds of host: (a) deficient in most phagocytic cells, (b) deficient in lymphocytes, and (c) normal. Looking along the time axis, you can see four distinct stages: (1) the first few hours, in which pathogen numbers fall because some are removed by macrophages resident in the tissues while others simply fail to survive the change to a new environment; (2) a period of growth which is checked, though not completely stopped, by mobile phagocytes together with complement, cytokines, and inflammatory responses, in the absence of which it may progress to death; (3) a period of a week or more in which pathogen numbers are brought down by adaptive responses which may in the long term result in (4) complete cure or, in the absence of this, persistence of some pathogens with the possibility of reactivation and relapse. We shall consider human immune deficiencies in more detail in Chapters 14 and 24; these unfortunate individuals have been most useful in defining exactly which parts of which immune system are responsible for controlling which infection.

11 Innate immunity

Also known by other names (e.g. natural, non-specific), the innate immune system comprises all those mechanisms for dealing with infection that are constitutive or 'built in', changing little with age or with experience of infection and, as already mentioned, traceable back to the earliest invertebrate forms of life (the synonym *natural* is often used, as a contrast to *adaptive* immunity; the term *non-specific* is rather out of date, since specificity in immunity is a relative matter). Though in some ways less sophisticated than adaptive immunity, innate immunity should not be belittled, since it has evidently protected thousands of species of invertebrates sufficiently to survive for up to 2 billion years—compared with the mere 500 million years of vertebrate evolution.

As emphasized in Chapter 10, all immune systems make use of molecular *recognition* elements, *disposal* mechanisms, and a *communication* system. In higher animals, these recognition and communication molecules may be either *cell-bound* or *soluble*. In the case of cell-bound molecules, their function is inseparable from that of the cell itself, and we speak of a 'cellular' type of immunity; an example would be the surface receptors by which phagocytic cells identify their prey (see below). In contrast, molecules that act freely in the extracellular compartment (e.g. complement, see below) are spoken of as 'humoral'. In the innate immune system, molecules of both types are involved, corresponding to the need to recognize and dispose of different types of pathogen, to promote inflammatory responses, which are of value in all types of infection, and to interact with the adaptive immune system. The principal cells and molecules are contrasted in Table 11.1, with some examples of their function and the appearance of some of the cells shown in Fig. 11.1.

Pattern recognition by the innate immune system

One of the key roles of the innate immune system is to distinguish between self and non-self, and where possible between self and *pathogen*. Such a distinction has been required since the evolution of multicellular life forms, which is why invertebrates, insects, and even plants have well developed innate recognition systems. In every case, recognition is mediated by the interaction of two sets of complementary molecules, as depicted in Fig. 11.2. Microorganisms have on

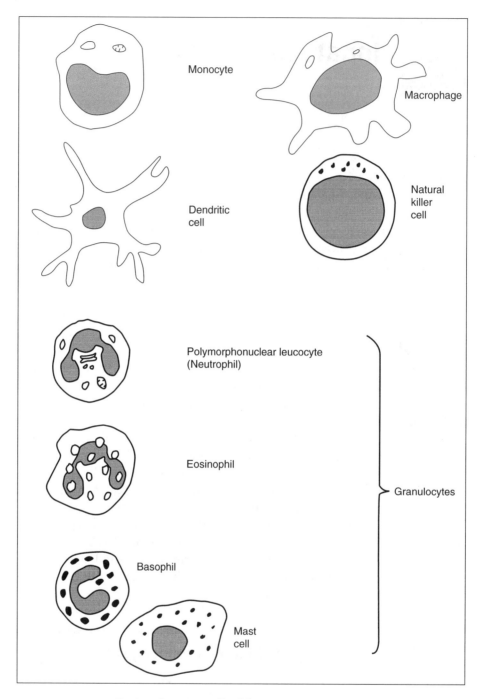

Fig. 11.1 Important cells of the innate immune system.

Table 11.1 The principal cells and molecules of innate immunity. Note the overlaps between the inflammatory response and the response to infection. +: major role; (+): relatively less important

	Anti-bacterial Anti-fungal	Anti-viral	Inflammatory	Interaction with adaptive imm.
Molecules				
Complement	+		+	(+)
Collectins	(+)		+	(+)
Other acute phase proteins	(+)		+	(+)
Interferons		+		+
Other cytokines			+	+
Cells				
Phagocytes	+	(+)	+	(+)
Dendritic cells				+
Mast cells			+	(+)
Natural killer cells	(+)	+		(+)

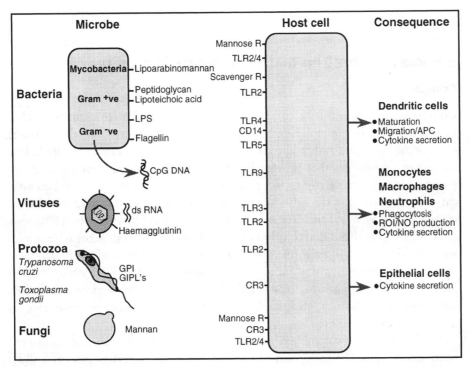

Fig. 11.2 Examples of cell-associated pattern recognition molecules and their microbial ligands. Note that most recognition events of whole organisms will involve more than one type of receptor acting in cooperation. Different host cells can also express distinct repertoires of recognition molecules. TLR: Toll-like receptor; GPI: glycosylphosphatidylinositol; GIPL's: glycosylinositolphospholipids; APC: antigen presenting cell function; ROI: reactive oxygen intermediates; NO: nitric oxide.

their surface certain 'pathogen-associated molecular patterns' (PAMP) which are either not present in the host or shielded in some way. Examples include lipopolysaccharide (Gram-negative bacteria), lipoteichoic acid (Gram-positive bacteria), mannans (fungal cell walls), double-stranded (ds) RNA (viruses), CpG DNA motifs (bacteria), and many others. These structures have been picked out for recognition because they are characteristic of microorganisms and often essential for their survival, and show minimal variation. Thus a microbe cannot evade recognition by simply mutating or eliminating them. The host structures that recognize them are called 'pattern-recognition molecules' and include many well-studied immune mediators such as complement as well as recently discovered ones such as the Toll-like receptor family (identified in mammals by their similarity to the Toll receptors used by the fruit fly *Drosophila* to recognize pathogens!). Pattern-recognition molecules may be either soluble (e.g. in blood) or membrane-bound (e.g. on phagocytes), and they are able to distinguish between, for example, Gram-negative bacteria and yeast, but without pinpointing the species of either. However, they trigger a sequence of events which not only attack the microorganism but also activate the adaptive immune system (see below and Chapters 15–19).

Soluble (humoral) mediators of innate immunity

Complement

Complement is the most striking example of a humoral innate immune mechanism. It is not a single molecule but a 'cascade system' of proteins that activate one another in series, rather like the blood clotting system (Fig. 11.3). Including the various inhibitors that prevent it getting out of control, there are over 30 plasma and cell surface complement components, the terminology being complicated by the fact that the full sequence of activation was not understood until quite recently, whereas the existence of the system was known in the 1880s—as soon as it was realized that antibodies needed another serum factor to 'complement' them in some of their functions. Only many years later was it understood that complement activation did not always require antibody, which is why the antibody-requiring pathway (restricted, like antibody, to vertebrates) is confusingly known as *classical*, and the others, found also in higher invertebrates, as *alternative* and *lectin-mediated*.

Though it appears complex, the complement system is actually amazingly economical, since the same central component, a major serum protein known as C3, can be activated in three different ways, and activation can lead to three different useful functions (Fig. 11.3). As always, its real value can be judged by the study of *deficiencies* and from these we learn that it matters most in bacterial infections (the same is true of *phagocytic cells* and *antibody*, as will be seen).

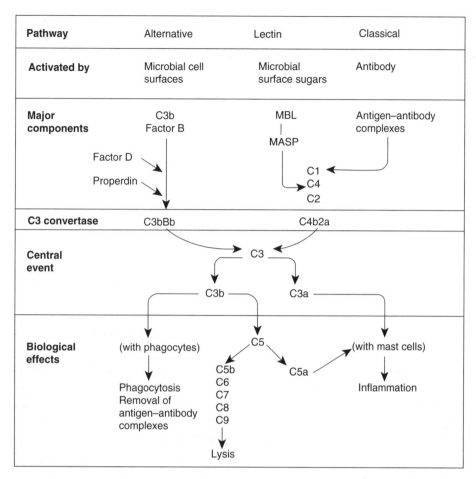

Fig. 11.3 The complement system, showing the three pathways of activation, the central role of C3, and the three biological effects. The many inhibitors by which activation is regulated are not shown.

Alternative pathway

The fundamental event in complement activation is the formation of a *C3 convertase* to split C3 into two fragments, C3b (large) and C3a (small), both of which have important functions. The convertase of the alternative pathway, known as C3bBb, involves three other serum proteins, factors B and D and properdin, as well as C3b itself, in a process that 'ticks over' slowly and harmlessly at host cell surfaces but is enormously enhanced at the surfaces of many bacteria, fungi, protozoa, and some viruses, so that large amounts of C3b are deposited there.

Lectin pathway

A second innate pathway of C3 convertase generation involves recognition of microbial surfaces by Mannose-binding lectin (MBL) and/or ficolins (see below).

These attach to repetitive patterns of mannose and other sugars, which are common in microbial but not mammalian cell surfaces, and activate the proteases MASP-1 and -2, which cleave two complement components C4 and C2, leading to the formation of the C3 convertase C4b2a, which acts similarly to C3bBb.

Classical pathway

The evolution of the antibody molecule (see Chapter 16) allowed a widening of the range of pathogens able to activate C3, through the ability of many antibodies to bind the complement component C1q which, together with C1r and C1s, induces the cleavage of C4 and C2. Thus C1q,r,s acts very much like MBL + MASP, except that not only sugar residues but potentially *any* pathogen-derived molecule can now activate the system. The classical pathway can also be activated by the acute phase protein CRP (see below).

Effector pathways

C3b is responsible for most of the benefits of complement activation. Bound to a pathogen, it can attach to *C3b receptors* on phagocytic cells and lead to *phagocytosis* (see below). C3b bound to a soluble antigen–antibody complex can attach the complex to (mainly) red cells and transport it to the phagocytes of the liver and spleen. C3b also cleaves C5 to C5b, which then associates with the complement components C6, C7, C8, and C9 to form the *membrane attack complex* which, by insertion into microbial membranes, particularly those of Gram-negative bacteria, leads to leakage and death by *lysis*. Finally, the small fragment C3a, together with C5-derived C5a, has its own role in promoting *inflammatory* reactions, mainly through binding to mast cells (see below).

Collectins and ficolins

MBL and other molecules that recognize sugar patterns unique to pathogens, or normally masked on healthy host cells, e.g. by sialic acid, are referred to as *collectins*, from their possession of a *coll*agen-like and a *lectin* domain. Other collectins include C1q itself, the surfactant proteins SP-A and SP-D found in the lung, and an ill-defined liver protein, CL-1. Ficolins possess an additional fibrinogen-like domain and can activate complement, but their exact role is not clear. Together they form part of a broader group of innate defence molecules called *defence collagens* sharing the property of recognizing pathogens and possibly some tumours (Fig. 11.4).

Acute phase proteins

One of the earliest detectable reactions to trauma or infection is the *acute phase response*. This is the name given to the inflammatory response leading to *fever* and other symptoms of illness including the appearance in the blood of a variety of 'acute phase' proteins, mostly made in the liver, in turn stimulated by cy-

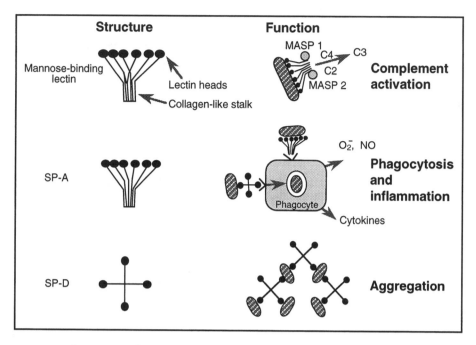

Fig. 11.4 Collectins and inflammation. Binding of pathogens by collectins can result in complement activation, phagocytosis, secretion of inflammatory mediators, and recruitment of inflammatory cells. SPA, SPD: important mediators of pulmonary inflammation, able to enhance/inhibit production by phagocytes of oxygen radicals, NO, and pro-inflammatory cytokines.

tokines secreted by phagocytes. From the list of these (Fig. 11.5) you can see that some are obviously useful in removing enzymes and other intracellular material released by tissue damage, but a few appear to have antibacterial properties too. This is especially true of *C-reactive protein* (CRP), a curious pentameric molecule ('pentraxin') that binds to the C polysaccharide of some streptococcal cell walls, activates complement, and promotes phagocytosis—somewhat like a primitive antibody molecule. The acute phase response is generated by a wide range of stimulants, and some of the individual components may not be needed in any one infection, but they flare up at the slightest sign of 'trouble'. For example, a raised level of CRP in the blood can be a useful early sign of an impending relapse in chronic diseases such as rheumatoid arthritis and some infections.

Cytokines

Most of the remaining mediators of innate immunity fall into the category of *cytokines*, already introduced in Chapter 10. As Table 11.2 shows, these have a wide range of activities but are essentially *communication* molecules, lacking in any direct pathogen recognition or disposal properties. Their effects overlap considerably, but can be roughly grouped into four categories, namely those

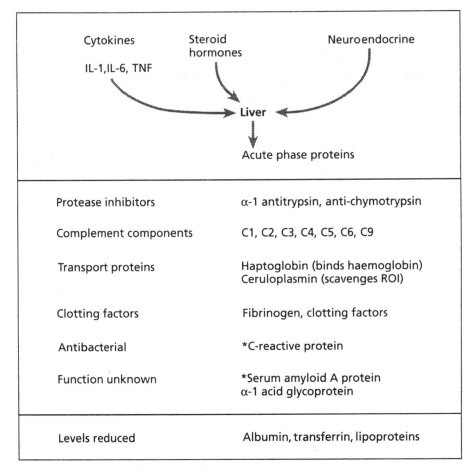

Fig. 11.5 During the acute phase response, the blood level of several proteins rises—some (*) by as much as 1000-fold. The response occurs within hours of injury or infection.

involved in the promotion of (1) *inflammatory* responses; (2) cell *differentiation and proliferation*; (3) cell *movement*; (4) *inhibition*, and (5) a special group of important antiviral molecules, the *interferons*. Note that cytokines, often the same ones, also play a major role in adaptive immunity; indeed they are responsible for most of the interactions between the two systems.

Interferons (IFN)

As with most cytokines, the IFN terminology is confusing because two of the three types of IFN, α and β, are very similar, whereas the third, γ, is a quite different molecule with many separate properties, notably that of activating macrophages to kill intracellular pathogens. However, their antiviral effects are the same: to induce an antiviral state in cells that otherwise might succumb to virus infection. Figure 11.6 illustrates the process by which this is brought about.

Table 11.2 Key cytokine groups of the innate immune system

	Cytokine	Cell source	Targets	Function
Inflammation	IL-1, IL-6 } TNF	Macrophages Dendritic cells, T cells	Hepatocytes endothelial cells hypothalamus macrophages, T cells, and B cells	Induction of acute phase response Recruitment of cells to inflammatory foci Induction of fever Phagocyte activation Proliferation of Ig-secreting B cells
Differentiation	IL-12, IL-18	Macrophages, Dendritic cells, Neutrophils	NK cells, T cells	Secretion of IFNγ by NK cells and T cells Increased T cell cytolytic activity Type 1 T cell differentiation
	IFNγ	NK, T cells	Macrophage	Activation
Proliferation	IL-15	Macrophages	NK cells and T cells	Proliferation
Cell movement	Chemokines e.g. IL-8, MIP-1α, RANTES, MCPs	Leukocytes	Multiple cell types	Recruitment of phagocytes to sites of infection Lymphocyte trafficking Lymphoid tissue development
Inhibition	IL-10, TGFβ	Macrophages, Dendritic cells, T cells	Macrophages, T cells	Inhibitors of macrophage activation Control of excessive inflammation Promote B cell growth Promote chronic fibrosis
Antiviral	Interferons	IFNα: macrophages IFNβ: fibroblasts IFNγ: NK, T cells	All cells	Induces antiviral state Increases MHC Class I expression Activates NK cell cytolytic activity

See also Appendix 2 and abbreviations list.

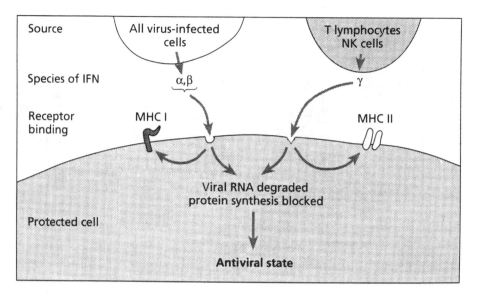

Fig. 11.6 The induction and activity of interferon molecules. The effects on major histocompatibility complex (MHC) cell-surface molecules are explained in Chapter 16.

Together with NK cells, IFNα and β are probably responsible for inhibiting many acute viral infections, and are also responsible for some of the symptoms, since it has been shown that large therapeutic doses of IFN and other cytokines can induce the fever, muscle pains, and general feeling of illness so typical of virus infections. Nevertheless they have come into use as therapeutic 'drugs' for certain virus infections as well as some tumours.

Cells of innate immunity

Phagocytic cells

Phagocytosis is the act of taking particulate matter into a cell, as opposed to taking in small molecules like water (pinocytosis). Many types of cell can phagocytose at times, but the specialized or 'professional' phagocytes of mammals are of two kinds: the large *macrophages* and the smaller *polymorphonuclear leucocytes* (PMN). These share many properties, but are designed to deal with different situations (Table 11.3). Cells with the essential features of macrophages may look different and are given different names in different sites (they used to be collectively known as the reticulo-endothelial system, a little-used term nowadays). Macrophages can present antigen to T cells, but there are also more specialized *antigen-presenting cells* (APC) in which phagocytosis has been reduced to the minimum necessary to induce adaptive responses in lymphocytes; these *dendritic*

Table 11.3 Phagocytic cells range from those with a predominantly scavenging role (top) to those mainly responsible for presenting small portions of phagocytosed material to lymphocytes (antigen-presenting cells, APC)

Cell type	Features	Functions
Polymorphonuclear leucocyte (PMN)	Short-lived (2 days), multi-lobed nucleus	Phagocytosis and killing of bacteria and fungi
Monocyte	In blood for 24 hours	Precursor of macrophage
Macrophage	Major phagocyte of tissues, long-lived (months, years)	Phagocytosis of damaged cells and molecules, foreign particles, microbes, etc.
Kupffer cell	Major phagocyte of liver	Clears blood of particles
Mesangial cell	Phagocyte of renal glomerulus	Removes complexes from glomerulus
Microglial cell	Phagocyte of brain	Phagocytosis
Dendritic cell (DC)	APC of lymphoid tissue	Presents antigen to naïve T cells
Langerhans cell	DC of skin (epidermis)	" " "

cells are described below, and will appear again when we consider the immune response in Chapters 17–19.

Phagocytosis is a complex, multi-step process by which a particle is 'eaten', prior to being killed and/or digested (Fig. 11.7). Note that a 'particle' may be anything from a speck of inhaled dust to an age-expired red cell or a nucleated cell that has self-destructed from the 'suicide' process known as apoptosis. As regards infectious organisms, phagocytosis is particularly effective against bacteria and fungi, and animals with defective phagocytes suffer from repeated infection with these types of pathogen. Often the phagocyte has to migrate through the tissues to find the pathogen, using *chemotactic* gradients of microbe-derived molecules or signals from other cells. Next, the phagocyte needs to attach the microbe to its membrane—the *recognition* stage, which may be by interaction with components of the microbial surface, often carbohydrate-based such as lipopolysaccharide or mannan (see Pattern Recognition, above), but which can be rendered more effective by the presence of *complement* or *antibody* on the microbe, because phagocytes also have receptors for these molecules on their surface; this process is known as *opsonization*. From then on, movements of the membrane and of intracellular vesicles guide the particle into the presence of powerful killing and digestive systems, reducing it to its molecular constituents for re-use or, alternatively, for expulsion from the body via sputum or faeces. In addition, small peptides of microbial origin may be transported to the cell surface by major

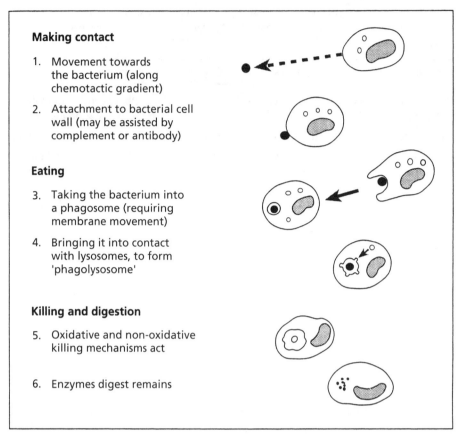

Making contact

1. Movement towards the bacterium (along chemotactic gradient)

2. Attachment to bacterial cell wall (may be assisted by complement or antibody)

Eating

3. Taking the bacterium into a phagosome (requiring membrane movement)

4. Bringing it into contact with lysosomes, to form 'phagolysosome'

Killing and digestion

5. Oxidative and non-oxidative killing mechanisms act

6. Enzymes digest remains

Fig. 11.7 Phagocytosis proceeds in steps, the whole process taking minutes or hours. Macrophages and PMN operate in much the same way, except that PMN are somewhat more potent in oxidative killing, and macrophages are more effective in dealing with long-lived parasites.

histocompatibility (MHC) molecules, to be 'presented' to T lymphocytes, as described in Chapter 17, and the act of phagocytosis may induce the release of inflammatory cytokines.

Not every phagocytic event proceeds to killing and digestion. Macrophages may need activation by IFNγ. Later you will read about pathogens that allow themselves to be taken into macrophages but not killed—an excellent long-term survival strategy for the pathogen. Some pathogens induce their own uptake by non-phagocytic cells, e.g. *Salmonella* into enterocytes.

Intracellular killing

Once inside the phagocyte, the majority of microbes are speedily killed. For this purpose, phagocytes have a selection of toxic molecules—some that derive from atmospheric oxygen ('oxidative killing') and others that do not require oxygen; the latter are needed where excess oxygen is not available, for example deep in

Table 11.4 Cells of the innate immune system contain numerous molecules toxic to parasites

Source	Molecules	Active against
PMN		
(1) In 'primary' granules	Lysozyme	Gram-positive bacteria
	Myeloperoxidase	Bacteria, fungi (with H_2O_2)
(2) in 'specific' granules	Defensins, BPI	Bacteria, fungi
	Lactoferrin	Bacteria (depletes iron)
Macrophage	As PMN but no myeloperoxidase	
	Nitric oxide	Intracellular pathogens
	Arginase	(depletes arginine)
Eosinophil	Cationic proteins	Worms (extracellular)
	Major basic protein	Worms (extracellular)
	Peroxidase	Worms (extracellular)
Natural killer cell	Perforins ⎤	Virus or bacteria
	Granzymes ⎦	infected cells
	Granulysin	Bacteria, fungi

Note that the granules of PMN are of two kinds, with different contents. Note also that the eosinophil granulocyte contains its own highly basic proteins, possibly designed to damage worms. BPI, bacterial permeability increasing factor, which binds to and inactivates endotoxins.

the tissues. Table 11.4 lists some of these non-oxidative molecules, and Fig. 11.8 summarizes the pathways by which the *reactive oxygen intermediates* and *nitric oxide* are formed; these are particularly prominent in PMN; their toxicity may be either direct or via induction of microbicidal proteases. To protect the phagocyte itself against these toxic compounds, they are packaged into vesicles called *lysosomes*, which can be steered into contact with the vesicles containing ingested material, which are known as *phagosomes* (see Fig. 11.7). Later you will see that some of the most awkward pathogens are those that resist all these killing mechanisms and take up long-term residence in phagocytes.

A second possibility, not so well understood, is that macrophages can sometimes stop the growth of microbes without killing them. This is sometimes seen with intracellular bacteria such as mycobacteria and legionella, and is referred to as bacteriostatic, in contrast to bactericidal; the mechanism is mainly one of starving the microbe of essential nutrients such as iron or tryptophan.

Dendritic cells

These cells have only been fully appreciated in the last decade or so but their importance in immunity is immense because they can be regarded as the primary interface between infectious organisms and the adaptive immune system. Their name is due to their shape, which is characterized by numerous long thin

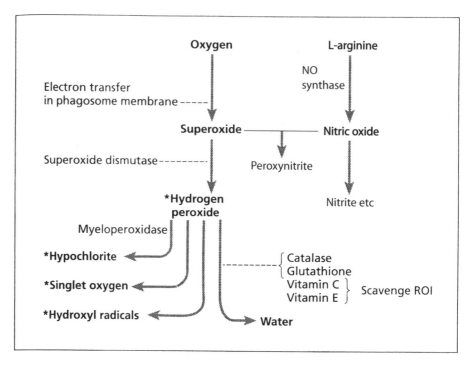

Fig. 11.8 Parallel and interacting metabolic pathways generate reactive oxygen (*ROI) and nitrogen intermediates by phagocytes. Note the presence of 'anti-oxidant' and scavenging molecules (right) to restrict the toxic activity of the ROI to the target (bacterium, fungus, etc.) without damage to the phagocyte itself. NO: Nitric oxide.

processes that project in all directions, giving them an enormous surface area at which to interact with both foreign material and other immunological cells, notably lymphocytes (Fig. 11.1). Ultimately derived from the bone marrow, dendritic cells show considerable heterogeneity in both appearance and function, and may in fact represent two separate lineages—one sharing an origin with NK cells and lymphocytes, the other with monocytes and macrophages.

Since their main function is in the initial 'presentation' of foreign material to lymphocytes at their surface, dendritic cells (e.g. in lymph nodes) specialize in recognition rather than phagocytosis. However, dendritic cells do have some phagocytic activity, particularly when immature in the periphery, and various pathogens are able to enter and survive in them; these include several viruses (measles, influenza, CMV, HIV) and some larger organisms (*Chlamydia, Leishmania*). Recognition by dendritic cells appears to involve much the same pattern-recognizing elements as those used by phagocytes, enabling dendritic cells to respond to a huge range of pathogenic material, from bacterial and protozoal surface molecules to bacterial DNA, viral RNA, and heat-shock proteins. To complete the impressive list of their activities, dendritic cells can secrete a variety of cytokines (IL-6, IL-12, IL-18, TNF, IFNα, β, γ), and in some infections, e.g. leishmaniasis, it is the dendritic cells rather than the macrophages that produce the transient burst of IL-12 which appears to be critical in initiating an effective cell-mediated immune response. In other infections they may be responsible for the IL-10 that *prevents* effective cell-mediated immunity.

Mast cells

Mast cells, prominent in the skin, around blood vessels, and in the gut, and the closely similar basophils in the blood, are of central importance in the *acute inflammatory response*, a series of changes designed to increase the supply of blood and its contents (PMN, complement, antibody, etc.) at local sites of trauma or infection (see below). Their function is to release the contents of their granules, which include histamine, leukotrienes, and other molecules that increase vascular permeability. This degranulation can be triggered by direct damage or under the influence of a special antibody (IgE); see Chapter 22 for an explanation of how this can lead to distressing *allergies*. Recent work has revealed that mast cells share a number of the features of dendritic cells, being able to some extent to take up foreign material, present antigens to lymphocytes, respond to some cytokines, and secrete others (e.g. TNF). Thus they are not just the 'explosive packages' of allergy but normally function in a more controlled way to initiate inflammation where required.

Lymphoid cells of innate immunity

This may seem a contradictory title, in view of what was said in Chapter 10 about the lymphocyte as the key cell of *adaptive* immunity, but certain cells of lymphocyte-like appearance display features typical of the innate system, most notably the natural killer cells.

Natural killer (NK) cells

These cells, sometimes known as large granular lymphocytes (LGL), were first identified by their ability to kill tumour cells which the host had not previously encountered—a 'natural' or *innate* type of killing in contrast to the adaptive antigen-specific type displayed by conventional cytotoxic T cells. They carry some of the cell surface markers of T cells (e.g. CD8) but not the classical T cell receptor. There is also an intermediate population of 'NK T cells' which do carry a restricted version of the T cell receptor (see Chapter 17).

The key features of NK cells are that they are much less restricted in their recognition than T cells and they respond rapidly—hours or days as compared to the days or weeks of conventional adaptive T cells. NK cells have been implicated in many immunological processes including tumour surveillance, regulation of haemopoiesis, bone marrow graft rejection, and the regulation of pregnancy. However, we know most about their role in infection, which is threefold:

(1) NK cells can have a direct effect by binding to the surface of some microorganisms, such as *Cryptococcus neoformans*. They are poorly phagocytic, but it is thought that the lytic machinery by which they kill tumour cells is released at the point of contact. It is fair to say that the evidence for this is largely derived from studies *in vitro*.

(2) Better understood are their effects on host cells: *lysis* of cells infected with intracellular pathogens, which is carried out by the release of NK granule contents such as the enzymes *perforin* and *granzymes* and the induction of apoptosis, and *killing* of intracellular pathogens by *granulysin*, a peptide with direct antimicrobial activity. The mechanism by which NK cells are triggered to lyse infected (or cancerous) but not normal host cells depends on a balance between two opposing forces: *activating* receptors that recognize target cell surface structures, including viral products, and give a 'kill' signal, and *inhibitory* receptors that recognize MHC Class I molecules and prevent killing. Only when MHC molecules are absent or altered (as in virus infection and some tumours) is the 'kill' signal allowed to predominate (Fig. 11.9).

(3) NK cells can also be stimulated by cytokines, such as phagocyte-derived IL-12 and IL-18, to release IFNγ which in turn activates the phagocytes to kill internalized pathogens such as bacteria (*Listeria*, *Salmonella*, *Mycobacterium*), protozoa (*Leishmania*, *Toxoplasma*), and some viruses (e.g. cytomegalovirus) (Fig. 11.10). The key point here is that the NK cells are a potent source of rapid IFNγ production (and cytotoxic activity), the rapidity being a typical innate immune feature.

Acute inflammation

We have already encountered inflammation in connection with complement, cytokines, and mast cells, but as Fig. 11.11 shows, there is more to it than this. Inflammation is one of the fundamental responses of the body to almost any kind of injury and a prerequisite for the healing process. Being a response to tissue damage, it is an inevitable part of the response to *pathogens*. Though its outward features, classically *rubor*, *calor*, *dolor*, *tumor* (redness, heat, pain, swelling), can be most unpleasant, its purpose is beneficial: to increase local blood supply and vascular leakage, allowing access to the affected site of blood, with its useful antimicrobial constituents—complement, phagocytes, lymphocytes, etc. Once infection is eliminated and damaged tissue removed, healing can begin. Note that Fig. 11.11 represents a great oversimplification; literally dozens of mediators are involved in both the induction and the down-regulation of inflammation, and over 50 genes have been identified which, if deficient or experimentally knocked out, cause inflammation to be prolonged, excessive, or even fatal. In addition, there are pathogens which are not easily eliminated. We shall return to this topic when we consider allergies and chronic inflammation in Chapter 22.

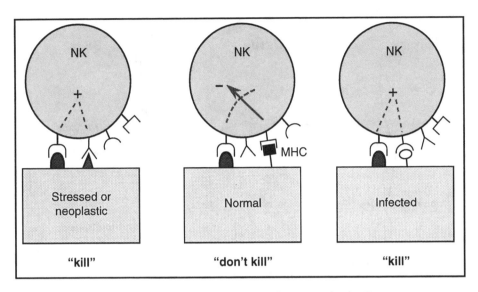

Fig. 11.9 Target recognition by NK cells. See text for details.

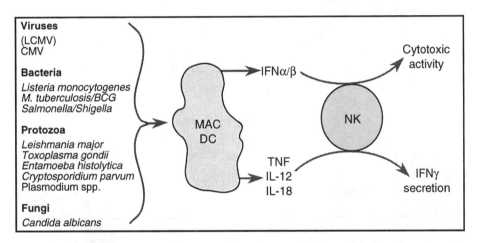

Fig. 11.10 NK cell activation by cytokines. Infections where IFN α/β production is dominant can favour cytotoxic activity (eg viruses) whereas IL-12/18 induced by bacteria, protozoa etc. also promotes IFNγ secretion.

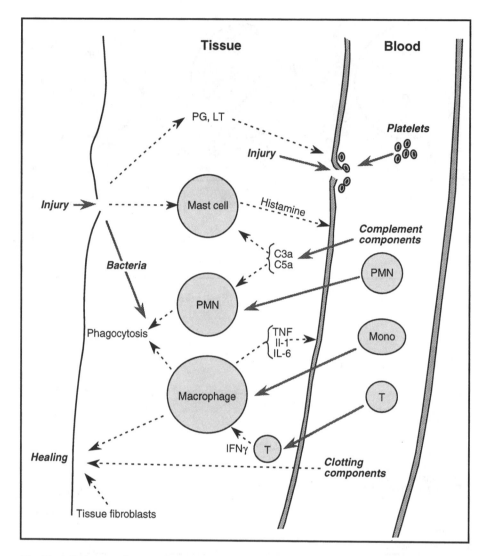

Fig. 11.11 Pathways of acute inflammation, showing the central role of vascular permeability. Solid arrows denote movement of cells/molecules; broken arrows denote effects on (1) blood vessel permeability: PG, prostaglandins; LT, leukotrienes; TNF, IL-1, IL-6, inflammatory cytokines; (2) mast cell and PMN activity: C3a, C5a, breakdown products of C3, C5; (3) phagocytosis of bacteria, also enhanced by antibody, not shown; (4) activation of macrophages: T, T lymphocyte; IFNγ, interferon gamma.

12 How pathogens escape innate immunity

Just as any parasite wishing to get into the body has to overcome the external defences (see Chapter 9), a pathogen wishing to survive in the body for more than a few hours will have to escape the powerful defence mechanisms of innate immunity, described in the previous chapter—phagocytes, complement, etc. The principal ways in which they do this are summarized in Table 12.1, in which they are classified according to the immune component they are designed to avoid. Another way to look at them is by analogy with an agent operating in enemy territory, and from *his* point of view. He has four main choices: to conceal his presence, to camouflage his appearance, to wear protective clothing, or to destroy enemy agents. In the case of pathogens, *concealment* includes getting inside host cells, as all viruses and many bacteria, fungi, and protozoa do, secreting impermeable barriers (some fungi), or inducing the host to form *cysts* or *granulomas* around the still-living pathogen (some bacteria and worms). 'Camouflage' strategies are usually aimed at preventing recognition, a particularly vital point where the lymphocytes of adaptive immunity are concerned (see Chapter 21) but also effective against recognition by complement and/or phagocytes, for example, the *capsules* that cover the cell wall of many of the most virulent bacteria (see below). 'Protective clothing' would correspond to the many devices pathogens have evolved to block or neutralize host attack, such as scavengers or inactivators of reactive oxygen intermediates. Finally, some pathogens directly attack host defences, bacterial toxins that destroy phagocytes and complement-splitting enzymes being good examples. The actual protective value of an individual escape mechanism is not always obvious, but if experimental deletion (e.g. by knocking out the gene concerned) leads to a reduction in virulence, one can be fairly sure of its importance to the pathogen. Note that many of the most successful survivors use more than one escape mechanism (c.f. *Leishmania*; see Table 12.1).

Avoiding complement

As well as blocking recognition by phagocytes, capsules can prevent activation of the alternative complement pathway. The thick peptidoglycan of Gram-positive

Table 12.1 Some examples of pathogen strategies for escaping the defence mechanisms of the innate immune system

Strategy	Examples
Intracellular habitat	Viruses: HIV, measles
	Bacteria: mycobacteria, *Brucella*
	Fungi: *Cryptococcus*
	Protozoa; *Leishmania, Toxoplasma*
Avoiding complement	
Capsules block activation	*Staphylococcus, Haemophilus*
LPS side chains block complement	Gram-negative bacteria
Enzymes destroy complement	
components	*Pseudomonas*
Mimicry of receptors for complement	Herpes simplex
Expulsion of membrane attack	
complex	*Leishmania*
Avoiding phagocytosis	
Killing of phagocytic cell	*Staphyloccocus, Streptococcus,*
	Listeria, Yersinia, Entamoeba
Production of capsules	*Strep. pneumoniae, Haemophilus*
Prevention of opsonization by	
antibody	Staphylococci (protein A)
Paralysis of uptake	*Yersinia*
Inhibition of chemotaxis	*Clostridia*, streptococci
Avoiding being killed in phagocyte	
Entry without activation	*Leishmania*
Inhibition of phagosome–lysosome	Mycobacteria, *Toxoplasma*
fusion and/or acidification	
Inhibition of reactive oxygen	Staphylococci (catalase)
intermediates	
Resistance to killing mechanisms	Mycobacteria, *Salmonella, Brucella*
Escape into cytoplasm	*Listeria, Shigella*
Inhibition of dendritic cells	HIV, CMV, *Leishmania*
Interference with cytokine network	
Mimicry of cytokine receptors	Pox viruses
Mimicry of inhibitory cytokines	Epstein–Barr virus
Inhibition of interferon	Adenovirus, vaccinia
Failure to induce interferon	Hepatitis B
Suppression of macrophage-	*Leishmania*, measles
derived cytokines	

membranes prevents the insertion of the C56789 complex, while *Leishmania* can expel the whole C56789 complex from its membrane, which then re-seals. Other anti-complement strategies include direct attack on the complement molecules themselves, by binding, cleaving, or expelling them, e.g. the elastase of *Pseudomonas* which destroys C3b and C5a, and the proteins of some viruses, bacteria, fungi, and protozoa which successfully mimic the inhibitors by which complement activation is normally regulated.

Avoiding phagocytosis

For bacteria, fungi, and protozoa, the phagocytic cell is their deadliest enemy, particularly when it is assisted by complement and/or antibody. Here pathogen survival strategies fall into three main categories: (1) prevent uptake; (2) if taken up, avoid being killed; (3) damage or destroy the phagocyte.

Preventing uptake

This can be further subdivided into the prevention of *recognition* and the *paralysis* of the uptake mechanism. The most striking example of the former is the bacterial *capsule*, usually polysaccharide, which covers up structures on the cell wall which the phagocyte would otherwise recognize. The protective effect of a capsule is illustrated by experiments in mice. Whereas about 10 capsulated pneumococci can kill a mouse, it takes 10 000 if the capsules are removed; in other words the capsulated bacterium is 1000 times more virulent. There is a fascinating molecule secreted by staphylococci, *protein A*, which inhibits IgG antibody from attaching to receptors and enhancing phagocytosis (see Chapter 16 for the molecular basis of this), and there are complement decoy proteins too (see above). Paralysis of the cytoskeletal reorganization required for the membrane movements of phagocytosis represents a most sophisticated approach; *Yersinia* (the plague bacterium) can do this, via injection of its own enzymes across the phagocyte membrane (so-called Type III secretion) which can inhibit the assembly of host actin into microfilaments.

Survival in the phagocyte

Some pathogens take a quite different approach, namely to let themselves be phagocytosed but resist the killing process. Often they are so successful that they are able to live unmolested within macrophages for months or years (PMN would have too short a lifespan to be suitable long-term hosts) and thus establish chronic infection. Mycobacteria (the tubercle and leprosy bacilli) are the classic example, but there are many others. Again, the mechanisms can be further subdivided, viz: (1) 'peaceful' entry into the phagocyte without triggering killing mechanisms (e.g. *Leishmania*); (2) escape from the phagosome into the cytoplasm, where killing mechanisms do not operate (e.g. *Listeria*); (3) inhibition of phagosome–lysosome fusion, notably by mycobacteria, the fungal pathogen *Histoplasma*, and the protozoon *Toxoplasma*; and (4) mopping up of microbicidal molecules, e.g. by the phenolic glycolipids of *M. leprae*, the catalase of *S.*

aureus, and the lipophosphoglycan of *Leishmania*, all of which counteract the respiratory burst and its toxic products. When we consider adaptive immunity (Chapter 19) you will see that these persistent intracellular pathogens constitute a real problem for the immune system. Activation of macrophages to overcome some of these inhibitory effects is one of the major roles of the T cell.

Damage to the phagocyte

The tendency of staphylococci and streptococci to cause cell necrosis is due to their *toxins*, the typical pus that fills a staphylococcal abscess being mainly composed of dead PMN and destroyed tissue cells. A more subtle approach is the induction of macrophage apoptosis ('cell suicide') as practised by *Yersinia*. Interestingly, some pathogens (e.g. *Chlamydia* and some viruses) *inhibit* apoptosis in order to ensure longevity of their host cell!

Avoiding natural killer cells

Look back to Chapter 11 to be reminded that NK cells are inhibited by the presence of MHC Class I molecules on the target cell. Some viruses (e.g. CMV) respond to this ingeniously by encoding an MHC Class I homologue which tricks the NK cell into inactivity while not engaging the attention of cytotoxic T cells, which respond to real MHC molecules (see Chapter 17). Other viruses (e.g. HIV, HSV) are able to infect and destroy NK cells.

Interference with dendritic cell function

Dendritic cells play a vital role in T cell activation, and some pathogens can inhibit this by directly infecting dendritic cells, leading to reduced maturation and cytokine release. In the case of HIV, infection of dendritic cells via a surface C-type lectin leads in turn to increased infection of T cells.

Interference with the cytokine network

Given the importance of cytokines in both natural and adaptive immunity, it is not surprising that pathogens have found ways to interfere with their function. There are now many different examples of how viruses specifically interfere with the immune system by encoding their own cytokines or cytokine inhibitors/ decoys. Among the most remarkable are the possession by the Epstein–Barr virus of a gene that codes for a molecule virtually identical to IL-10, a cytokine that inhibits the production of several other cytokines (an example of *mimicry*), and the possession by pox viruses of a molecule similar to the soluble TNF receptor, which can 'mop up' the natural cytokine (see Table 21.2). Inhibition of interferon induction or activity is another obviously useful strategy for viruses. In other cases the same result is achieved by stimulating the over-production by the host of inhibitory cytokines such as TGFβ and IL-10.

The role of vectors

Biting insects are an important means of transmission for several tropical pathogens (malaria, leishmaniasis, dengue, etc.) and may also help them survive. For example, the saliva of sandflies (the vector of *Leishmania*) inhibits macrophages and T cells, and can induce inhibitory host factors such as PGE2 and IL-10. While not actually pathogen-derived, this local immunosuppression protects the pathogen in the earliest stages of infection.

Taking all these evasion strategies into consideration, one can appreciate that, powerful as innate immunity is, the battle does not always go its way. It is generally assumed that the success of these ingenious pathogens was the driving force for the evolution of adaptive immunity, to be described in Chapters 15–19.

13 Disease due to innate immunity

Referring back to Chapter 8, you will be reminded that disease, that is, *pathology*, is sometimes due to the pathogen alone (e.g. cytopathic viruses; toxins), but can also be produced by the immune system. Here we will discuss the ways in which innate immune mechanisms can lead to pathology; the much more diverse ways in which adaptive immunity can do this are described in Chapters 22 and 23.

Both the phagocytic cells and the complement system have tremendous potential for damaging host cells, but fortunately they are normally only triggered by foreign materials, and usually most of their destructive effects are focused on the surface of these, or in the safe environment of the phagolysosome (but see below). However, there is one class of microbial molecule which can cause havoc in the immune system, and outside it, and this is *endotoxin*, the cell-wall lipopolysaccharide (LPS) of some but not all Gram-negative bacteria (Table 13.1), which is responsible for many cases of *sepsis*. Gram-positive bacteria lack endotoxin, though they do have toxins (e.g. the TSST-1 of *Staphylococcus aureus*) whose effects depend on over-stimulation of T lymphocytes (see Chapter 17).

Three related terms need to be distinguished: *septicaemia* denotes the presence of bacteria in the blood; *sepsis* refers to the failure of one or more organs caused by over-reaction to infection; *septic shock* describes the most severe situation with vascular collapse, which carries a mortality of up to 50%. For example, septicaemia, leading to septic shock, is one of the feared complications of *meningococcal meningitis*.

Endotoxin-induced pathology

The number of systems affected by this innocuous-looking molecule (Fig. 13.1) is quite remarkable (Fig. 13.2). Some of these, for example the clotting system, are not strictly immunological, but the comment of a famous American immunologist that 'when we sense lipopolysaccharide, we are likely to turn on every defence at our disposal' makes the point.

The effects of LPS, particularly those on the vascular system, appear to be

Table 13.1 The major endotoxin-containing bacteria

E. coli	*Klebsiella*
Proteus	*Neisseria*
Bordetella	*Salmonella*
Pseudomonas	*Shigella*
Haemophilus	

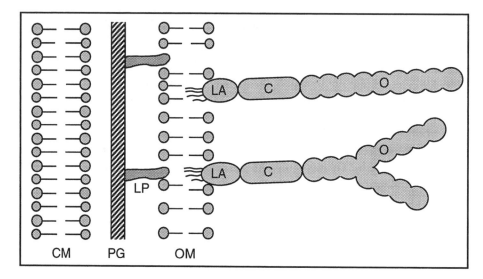

Fig. 13.1 Two LPS molecules in the wall of a Gram-negative bacterium. CM: Cell membrane; PG: Peptidoglycan; OM: Outer membrane; LP: Lipoprotein; LA: Lipid A; C: Core polysaccharide; O: O polysaccharide side chains (O antigens).

mainly due to the induction of excessive cytokine secretion by macrophages, mediated by complex signalling systems (Fig. 13.3). TNFα, IL-1 and IL-12 are the major cytokines involved. In a classic experiment it was shown that a neutralizing antibody against the cytokine TNFα was all that was needed to protect baboons from the otherwise lethal drop in blood pressure ('endotoxin shock') following a large injection of *E. coli*, and the same approach has been tried in patients with septic shock. This seemed to offer an alternative to the use of antibodies against endotoxin itself, which have proved very hard to produce. However, by its very nature, septic shock is a complex and multi-component syndrome, and the effects of cytokine-based intervention have been generally poor. This is due in part to the fact that when patients present to the physician they are already well into the cascade of cytokine production and at this stage blocking a single cytokine is too late. This is supported by the pre-clinical studies in experimental animals where such treatments need to be given at or before the time of infection in order to have any therapeutic effect. However, there is

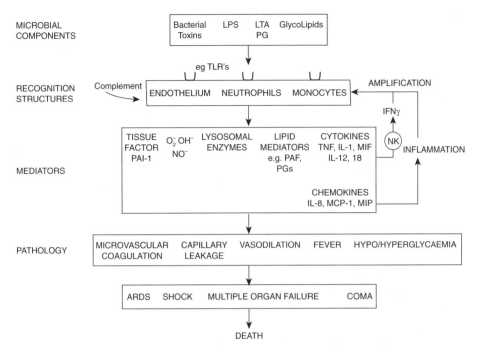

Fig. 13.2 Endotoxin and similar molecules activate numerous defence mechanisms which, if pushed to excess, can have serious and even fatal consequences. For abbreviations see text.

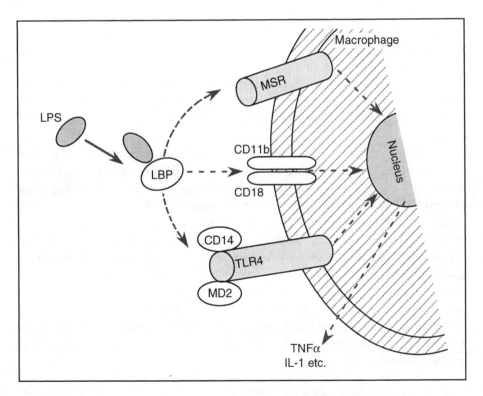

Fig. 13.3 Recognition of LPS occurs primarily via interaction of LPS: LBP with CD14: TLR-4: MD2 but other receptors such as MSR and CD11b/CD18 can also be involved. LBP: LPS-binding protein; TLR4: Toll-like LPS receptor; CD14: LPS receptor; MD2: TLR4 co-factor; MSR: macrophage scavenger receptor.

evidence that some degree of self-regulation occurs naturally, in the form of cytokine inhibitors (e.g. TNF and IL-1 receptor antagonists), inhibitory cytokines (e.g. IL-10), complement inhibitors, anti-inflammatory corticosteroids etc. Note that pathogens other than bacteria share the property of inducing high levels of inflammatory cytokines; these include mycobacteria, yeasts, and the malaria parasite.

Another target of endotoxin is the complement system (alternative pathway, see Fig. 11.3). Massive complement activation, with the consequent inflammation, can damage small blood vessels and this, together with the accumulation of PMN and perhaps the direct effects of TNF, can lead to leakage of fluid into the lung alveoli—a condition known as *adult respiratory distress syndrome* (ARDS), one of the most dreaded complications of severe injury and/or infection. Widespread blood clotting (*disseminated intravascular coagulation*, DIC) and overactivation of the fibrinolytic pathway, coupled to the lowered blood pressure and decreased oxygen supply, lead to the vital organ failure of *septic shock*.

At a more benign level, many people have experienced the effects of small doses of endotoxin following injection of killed *Salmonella typhi* organisms—the typhoid vaccine—and with a little practice one can distinguish for oneself the feeling of illness due to TNF and/or IL-1 (e.g. Gram-negative intestinal infections) from that due to interferon (e.g. severe influenza). It is suspected that the endotoxin of *Bordetella pertussis* may be to blame for the neurotoxicity attributed to the whooping-cough vaccine, though this whole field is controversial (see Chapter 27). There may also be a transient inflammatory response following treatment with antibiotics that disrupt large numbers of bacteria and release endotoxin—though other similar reactions may be allergic in nature, for example the Mazzotti reaction that can follow the killing of some worms.

In addition to the examples of endotoxin-induced pathology, there is great interest in the idea of inhibiting the dangerous complications of a wide range of diseases by interrupting cytokine pathways. Thalidomide, a drug with a tragic clinical history, turns out to be a potent and relatively selective inhibitor of TNF production and is being tested for preventing TNF-mediated pathology and wasting in leprosy and HIV, respectively. The recent successful use of anti-TNF antibodies to reduce the severity of arthritis points to the potential benefits of such an approach in inflammatory as well as infectious diseases. However, long-term interference with the cytokine system may come with a price, as a few patients receiving these antibodies now show an increased risk of reactivating latent *M. tuberculosis*, reminding us that TNF is also an essential component of the protective innate response. Figure 13.4 illustrates some possible approaches to these problems.

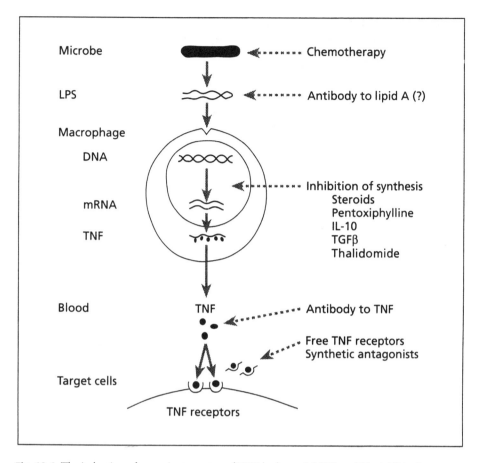

Fig. 13.4 The induction of excessive amounts of TNF by bacterial LPS could be inhibited at several levels. Similar strategies can be designed for other cytokines.

Polymorphs, mast cells, and complement

As mentioned in Chapter 11, much of the destructive power of phagocytes—particularly polymorphs—is due to the intracellular production of *reactive oxygen intermediates* (ROI) derived from atmospheric oxygen. Unfortunately, whenever large numbers of polymorphs are activated, there is the risk of ROI escaping and damaging the surrounding tissues. It is thought that in some degenerative diseases, especially of blood vessels, the damage is caused by ROI, which is why chemists' shops are full of pills containing 'antioxidants' such as vitamin C, vitamin E, seleniums, etc. Whether these really do any good has never been critically established, but certain lipids found in fish oil do have mild anti-inflammatory activity.

The activation of complement, normally restricted to the vicinity of pathogens by inhibitors (see Chapter 11), may also lead to tissue damage in extreme cases; examples are endotoxin shock (see above) and *immune complex disease*—though the latter is initiated by antibody (see Chapter 22). Complement activation may also cause damage when one of the natural inhibitors is absent, as in the disease *hereditary angioedema* (see Chapter 14).

For completeness we should mention the curious phenomenon of *anaphylactoid* reactions, in which mast cells are triggered by chemical means (e.g. some radiological contrast media) rather than as usual by antibody, and discharge their contents (histamine, etc.) resulting in violent and dangerous local inflammation.

14 Immunodeficiency I: primary defects of innate immunity

It would be surprising if such a complex collection of cells and molecules as the immune system did not occasionally malfunction. In fact, serious *immunodeficiency* is fairly rare (about 3 per 100000 of the UK population, rising to 1 in 1500 if the most minor defects are included) but remains an important cause of increased susceptibility to infection. Almost any part of the immune system may be affected. It may be faulty from the start because of a congenital defect (*primary immunodeficiency*) or it may be damaged later in life for a variety of reasons (*secondary immunodeficiency*). In this chapter we will concentrate mainly on immunodeficiency affecting the innate immune system; defects of adaptive immunity, which are considerably more common (see Fig. 14.1), are dealt with in Chapter 24.

Genetics of primary immunodeficiency

Primary defects are *genetic* abnormalities, usually single recessive mutations, that affect the proper development of some component. They may be *inherited* if the mutation is in a gene present in the germ-line. Two patterns of inheritance can be distinguished, depending on which chromosome is affected.

1 X-linked. The gene lies on the X chromosome, but being recessive it does not cause symptoms in females, who will also have a normal gene on the other X chromosome except in the rare situation where both parents carry the defect. However 50% of male offspring, with only one X chromosome, will be affected. This is the same 'sex-linked' inheritance as seen in haemophilia: mother to male offspring.

2 Autosomal recessive. The gene lies on some other chromosome. Heterozygotes are likely to be normal *carriers*, but homozygotes (both parents being carriers) will be affected.

Since more than one mutation per gene is possible, and sometimes two or more versions of the same gene can coexist in the population (polymorphism), the results can vary from severe losses of some important immune function to quite mild deviations from the normal. Correspondingly some patients are

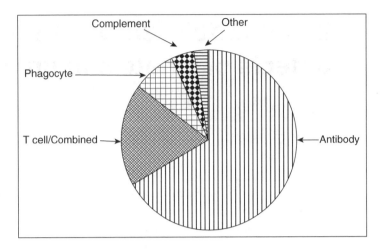

Fig. 14.1 Comparative frequency of the major immune deficiency syndromes.

dramatically prone to infection from birth while other defects pass unnoticed except in special circumstances, and even patients with the same defect may display varying levels of susceptibility to infection. Infections in immunodeficient patients include not only the common pathogens but also organisms that are not pathogenic at all in normal individuals—the so-called *opportunistic* infections. In addition, there is a significantly increased risk of malignancy and autoimmunity.

Ironically, the study of immunology has benefited greatly from immune deficiencies, which are often the best guide to the real role of a particular immune component. Further knowledge has come from animals, either from naturally occurring defects or, most informative of all, from the deliberately engineered elimination of particular genes by the so-called 'knock-out' technology. In general, it has been found that the absence of most components affects only resistance to infection (and some tumours), though it is of course possible that some of the defects we do *not* see are in fact incompatible with normal fetal development for other reasons.

Primary defects of innate immunity

The most common primary defects affecting the innate system are those involving complement and phagocytic cells, which give rise to quite characteristic patterns of infection (Table 14.1).

Table 14.1 Common infections in defects of innate immunity

Defect	Most frequent infections			
	Viruses	Bacteria	Fungi	Protozoa and worms
Complement				
C3		Staph., strep. *Pseudomonas*		
C5–9		*Neisseria*		
Cytokines				
Interferon IL-12	Respiratory	Mycobacteria		
Phagocytic cells		Staph., strep. *Pseudomonas*	*Candida* *Aspergillus*	
CGD		Staph., *E. coli*		
MPO			*Candida*	
NK cells	Herpes			
Other				
Cystic fibrosis		Staph., *Haemophilus* *Pseudomonas*		
*Splenectomy		*S. pneumoniae* *N. meningitidis*		*Babesia*

* Probably includes an element of adaptive (antibody) deficiency.

Complement defects

Several patterns of complement deficiency can be distinguished.

1 Reduced levels of C1s esterase inhibitor, resulting in overactivity of the 'classical' pathway and reduction in levels of C2 and C4, with recurrent inflammatory attacks and swelling of mucosal tissue which may lead to laryngeal or intestinal obstruction. This condition, the commonest defect involving complement, is known as *hereditary angioedema.*

2 Low or absent levels of C1, 2, or 4, which lead to difficulty in clearing antigen–antibody complexes from the circulation, and are a frequent feature of the disease systemic lupus erythematosus, in which the kidney and other organs are damaged by the deposition of immune complexes (see Chapter 22).

3 Low or absent levels of C5–9, which predispose to serious infections with bacteria of the *Neisseria* class such as disseminated gonorrhoea and meningococcal meningitis. This increased susceptibility suggests that in this group of infections, the formation of a lytic membrane-attack complex (see Chapter 11) is of real importance in clearing the infection. It is surprising that the great

majority of bacterial infections are *not* worsened by these defects, emphasizing the importance of phagocytosis rather than lysis in most infections.

4 Survival in the absence of the central component C3 is, as one might expect, extremely rare, though it has been reported.

Other soluble molecules

Deficiency of the mannose-binding lectin, MBL, can lead to severe infections in children. MBL is a member of the collectin family (see Chapter 11) with a role in complement activation, phagocytosis, and inflammation, and considerable individual variations exist in MBL levels, reflected in different susceptibility to infection, particularly in young children. In addition there are mutations that affect the structure of the molecule, or that lead to its complete absence; in such children severe recurrent bacterial and fungal infections occur. Low MBL levels in adults are less serious except when adaptive immunity is also defective, as for example in AIDS (see Chapter 25).

Cytokines

The most commonly reported defects are of IL-12 and IFNγ and of the IFNγ receptor. IFNγ receptor deficiency leads to a predisposition to infection with intracellular pathogens, such as atypical mycobacteria (including BCG), salmonella, and *Listeria*, affected children often dying before the age of 10. IFNα deficiency is associated with repeated viral respiratory infections. Interestingly, absence of the chemokine receptor CCR5 causes significant *resistance* to HIV infection, this molecule being also the macrophage 'second receptor' for the virus.

Cellular defects

Defects in myeloid cell development

(1) In reticular dysgenesis there is bone marrow stem-cell failure with an almost complete absence of blood monocytes and neutrophils plus reduced numbers of lymphocytes and a rapidly fatal outcome.

(2) Neutropenia (low or absent neutrophil numbers) may be congenital or cyclical. In the latter, blood neutrophil levels oscillate periodically with often a 3-week cycle and recurring bouts of oropharyngeal and/or skin infection.

Defects in myeloid cell function
Phagocytic cells

(1) Inability to respond to chemotactic stimuli and move through the tissues towards an inflammatory site ('lazy leucocyte').

(2) Leucocyte adhesion deficiency. Inability to attach to vascular endothelium as a prelude to migrating from blood to tissue. Two different defects have been identified, both affecting molecules involved in leucocyte–endothelial cell interaction. As a result blood leucocyte levels are high and bacterial and fungal infections are common.

(3) Chediak–Higashi syndrome. Failure of phagosomes to fuse with lysosomes (see also natural killer cells, below).

(4) Chronic granulomatous disease. Defect of one of the four components of NADPH oxidase involved in the oxidative killing pathway (see Chapter 11), leading to prolonged infection and abscess and granuloma formation with bacteria such as *Staphylococcus aureus* and fungi such as *Aspergillus* which would normally be killed by the oxidative burst. Catalase-positive microbes are the most dangerous, because catalase destroys hydrogen peroxide; catalase-negative organisms such as *Strep. pneumoniae* produce their own hydrogen peroxide, which to some extent overrides the cell's NADPH oxidase defect. The disease can be easily diagnosed by an *in vitro* test on the patient's neutrophils (NBT test). In addition to antibiotics, treatment with IFNγ has proved effective.

(5) Deficiency of myeloperoxidase and other enzymes, with somewhat similar results to the above.

(6) Neutrophil specific granule deficiency: self-explanatory and extremely rare.

Natural killer cells

In the Chediak–Higashi syndrome, the intracellular movement of lysosomes is abnormal, resulting in giant non-functional lysosomes. NK cell and neutrophil-mediated killing is affected (and in some cases that of cytotoxic T cells, see Chapter 19).

Total absence of NK cells is associated with repeated infection with the herpes viruses HSV and CMV.

Cystic fibrosis

In this condition, abnormally sticky mucus prevents the normal functioning of the muco-ciliary escalator (see Chapter 9). Though not strictly an immune defect, cystic fibrosis is one of the commonest causes of repeated bacterial lung infections in children.

Treatment

The treatment of both innate and adaptive immunodeficiency syndromes is discussed in Chapter 24. In the case of the innate defects, replacement therapy is usually not practicable and management relies on treatment of infections, e.g. with antibiotics.

Secondary immunodeficiency

Most adult immunodeficiencies fall into this category, and taken together they are far commoner than the primary deficiencies discussed above. The causes range from malnutrition (the commonest worldwide) to infections such as HIV, tumours, drugs, X-irradiation, trauma, and diseases such as diabetes. It is not always possible to identify which immune component is affected, but since there is usually an element of lymphocyte (adaptive) involvement, they will be discussed in more detail in Chapter 25.

Tutorial 2

You have now learned something about the immune system, and quite a lot about innate immunity. Write specimen sets of headings for the following essay questions, concentrating as before on presenting them in a logical and interesting sequence.

1. 'Because the phagocytes have retained the primitive property of taking up food, they can act as destroyers of parasites. They seem, therefore, as the bearers of Nature's healing power . . .' (Metchnikoff 1884). Was Metchnikoff right?

2. '. . . the mixture becomes clear and red within minutes . . . the corpuscles of this rabbit have thus become sensitive to their own alexine under the influence of a foreign clumping substance from a guinea pig treated with injections of the blood' (Bordet 1898). What did Bordet mean by alexine? What was the clumping substance? Discuss the significance of Bordet's finding.

3. Cytokines are the hormones of the immune system. Discuss.

4. Recognition of foreignness; the more specific the better. Discuss.

5. Oxygen is the cell's best friend and worst enemy. Discuss.

6. What is 'natural' about natural killer cells?

Some ideas for you to consider.

1. This is from Metchnikoff's classic paper in which he described phagocytes eating fungal particles in a transparent water flea. Fundamentally, he was right; the phagocyte is probably the single most valuable anti-microbial element. But it is of course not the only one! In Metchnikoff's day, scientists were sharply divided into proponents of cells as the major defence mechanism, and champions of humoral factors such as antibody. Since both are important, frequently acting together (as proposed by Sir Almroth Wright in 1903), the debate eventually died out. Amazingly enough, it was not until the 1950s and 1960s that lymphocytes were proved to be involved in immunity at all!

2. Alexine was the original name for complement, and the clumping substance was *antibody*. Put into modern language, what Bordet was saying was that

injecting rabbit blood (i.e. red cells, a safer substitute for bacteria) into a guinea pig induced the formation of antibody against the red cells, which would clump them in a test tube. But in order to destroy (i.e. lyse) the red cells, something from normal rabbit serum is needed, namely, complement—actually a series of interacting proteins that can punch holes in membranes. This experiment illustrates perfectly the distinction between innate (complement) and adaptive (antibody) immunological molecules.

3. This is a useful analogy, emphasizing the fact that cytokines are small soluble molecules that convey instructions from cell to cell. Thus thyroid-stimulating hormone (TSH) 'tells' the thyroid to secrete thyroxine; the cytokine interferon gamma (IFNγ) 'tells' macrophages to secrete tumour necrosis factor; the 'target' cells carry receptors for TSH and IFNγ, respectively. However, TSH is made only in the pituitary, and acts only on the thyroid, whilst INFγ is made by several cell types (T cells, NK cells), acts on many cells, and produces many different effects. Also it exerts most of its activity on cells in the immediate vicinity, whereas with TSH it is the blood level that matters, since pituitary and thyroid cells cannot make direct contact. Note that there are molecules such as erythropoietin that are often classified as both hormones and cytokines, so the definitions are not really precise, and either a 'yes' or a 'no' answer to the question could be justified, provided the facts were right and the case well argued.

4. It depends what you mean by better. For a rapid response to, for example, bacterial infection, the more cells that can be involved the better, which means that some cells must recognize more than one type of bacterium. Phagocytes and (for viruses) NK cells do this, i.e. they are non-specific. But for developing memory, to deal progressively better with infections that are not got rid of rapidly and recur frequently, it is more economical for only a few cells to respond initially and then build up their numbers, leaving others to deal with infections with other microbes. Lymphocytes do this, i.e. they are specific. Each approach has its strengths and weaknesses, and higher animals seem to require both for healthy life. The analogy with a police force (street patrol versus detectives) is useful: try and imagine a force restricted to one or the other type of officer.

5. A typical overstatement but it contains a germ of truth. The earliest organisms are thought to have developed in the absence of oxygen, and even today some, notably the anaerobic bacteria, are killed by it. The evolution of electron-transport chains using oxygen permitted the emergence of aerobic respiration, but even aerobic cells are susceptible to the toxic effects of reactive oxygen intermediates (ROI)—superoxide, hydrogen peroxide, hydroxyl radicals, singlet oxygen. In phagocytic cells, these are generated following phagocytosis and kill the majority of bacteria and fungi. The cell itself is protected by catalase, glutathione, etc., but escaping ROI are thought to be responsible for degenerative diseases of blood vessels, lung, brain, etc.

6. Natural killer (NK) cells are so named because, like all other components of the innate ('natural') immune system, they act rapidly, use germ-line encoded receptors, and as far as we know do not display memory. By contrast the cytotoxic T lymphocytes, which kill in the same way but carry specific receptors and develop memory, might be called 'adaptive killer cells'. The distinction between innate and adaptive immune mechanisms is not just for the convenience of teachers and students, but represents two fundamentally different ways of going about the job of recognizing and disposing of foreign invaders, in this case intracellular viruses.

15 Adaptive immunity: introduction

Compared to the numerous elements of the innate immune system just described, adaptive immunity merely added one new type of cell—the *lymphocyte*. But the possibilities inherent in this cell are so extraordinary and apparently endless that the adaptive immune system ranks second only to the brain in scope and flexibility. It is called 'adaptive' because of the way it allows both species and individuals to 'tailor-make' their own set of recognition molecules, adapted to the microbes they actually encounter, rather than simply relying on a fixed set and hoping that one or other of them will succeed. The analogy has already been made of the immune system as a kind of army, but another good parallel is with the *police*: if innate immunity is like the policeman on the street, watching out for obvious villains of whatever kind, adaptive immunity is like the detective branch, trained to spot each individual criminal, however elusive, track him down, and keep him on file for the future. In immunological language, the system displays *high specificity* and *memory*.

The lymphocyte

Besides specificity and memory, two other properties distinguish lymphocytes from other immunological cells: the ability to *recirculate* throughout the body and the ability to *proliferate* and *differentiate* (that is, to *respond*) on demand. Table 15.1 brings out the essential differences between lymphocytes and phagocytic cells.

There are two different kinds of lymphocyte, known as B and T because of their origin from the *bone* marrow and *thymus*, respectively (by a lucky chance, the B cells of birds are derived from an organ near the cloaca called the *bursa* of Fabricius). Put very simply, B lymphocytes (or B cells as they are often called) are responsible for 'policing' the extracellular body spaces—blood, tissue fluids, etc.—while T cells monitor the intracellular compartments, a more difficult task. However, as you will see (Chapters 18 and 19) they frequently interact with each other and with components of the innate immune system. Furthermore, once lymphocytes have carried out their recognition step, phagocytic cells, complement, etc. are still responsible for much of the disposal of the foreign material. Table 15.2 sums up the main differences between B and T cells.

Table 15.1 Lymphocytes differ from phagocytic cells such as macrophages in four main respects, which together maintain the flexibility of the adaptive immune system

1. They *recirculate* through the blood, tissues, and lymphoid organs, waiting to encounter foreign molecules (or *antigens*).

2. They are individually *specific* for the antigens they recognize. This is due to the possession of antigen-specific surface receptors.

3. When they recognize 'their' antigen, they *respond* by proliferating and switching on a particular function (e.g. cytotoxicity; secretion of antibody or cytokines).

4. Once they have functioned, some of them remain for years as *memory* cells, with the capacity for faster and larger future responses.

Table 15.2 B and T lymphocytes differ in several important respects

	B lymphocytes	T lymphocytes
Origin	Bone marrow (in fetal life the liver, in birds the bursa)	Thymus (stem cells from bone marrow)
Recognition molecules	Antibody (immunoglobulin)	T cell receptor
Secreted product(s)	Antibody	Cytokines
Disposal mechanisms	Antibody (leading to phagocytosis, lysis)	Some T cells are cytotoxic, others activate phagocytes
Mainly effective against	Extracellular infection	Intracellular infection

The lymphoid system

This term is used to describe the total mass of lymphocytes in the body, some of which are at any given time recirculating through the blood, while others are in scattered solid organs such as the lymph nodes, spleen, tonsils, etc. (Fig. 15.1). It is estimated that, if put together, the lymphocytes of a normal adult would occupy a space about the size of a football. Lymphoid organs are conventionally classified as *primary* or *secondary*, the former being the sites of lymphocyte formation and the latter the sites in which they carry out their function of recognizing and responding to foreign material. Secondary lymphoid organs are situated in strategic positions where infectious organisms are likely to be found: lymph nodes for the tissues; the spleen for the blood; tonsils and adenoids for the nose and throat; Peyer's patches and other lymphoid collections for the gut. A simple test for the difference between primary and secondary lymphoid organs is that if a primary organ fails to develop, the corresponding population of lymphocytes

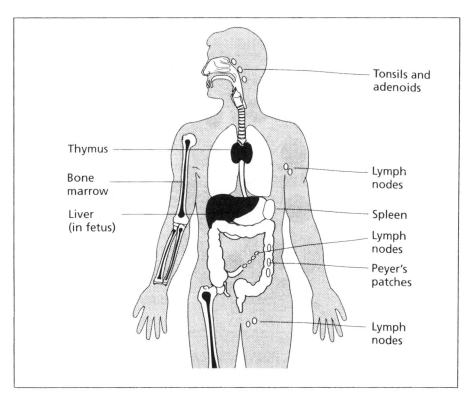

Fig. 15.1 The location of the major lymphoid organs: *left*, primary; *right*, secondary.

is permanently missing; this does occasionally happen (see primary immunodeficiency, Chapter 24).

Within the lymphoid organs, B and T lymphocytes are concentrated in particular sites, mainly determined by the resident antigen-presenting cells (APC) in the organ. Different cells 'present' foreign molecules (the word *antigen* is used for molecules that lymphocytes recognize, as will be explained in Chapters 16 and 17), and the flow of lymphocytes through the lymphoid organs is arranged so that each type encounters the right APC as well as other lymphocytes with which it needs to interact. Figure 15.2 illustrates the general design of a lymph node.

Recirculation

The ability to recirculate through the tissues, the lymphoid organs, and the blood is a fundamental part of lymphocyte function, enabling any lymphocyte eventually to make contact with an antigen, no matter where it is. Recirculation follows two patterns: (1) a random 'tick-over' that goes on all the time, from blood to tissues to lymph and back to blood, and (2) an enhanced and focused attraction

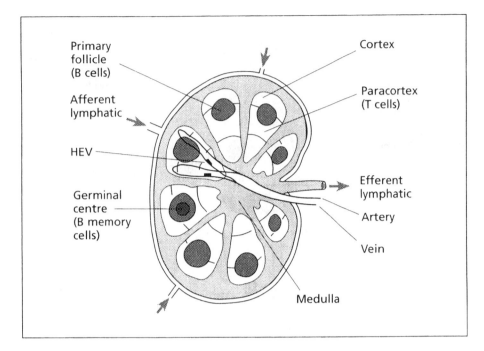

Fig. 15.2 The structure of a typical lymph node, showing the compartmentalization of B and T lymphocytes. Only one vascular loop is shown. HEV is a high endothelial venule, the site of lymphocyte emigration from blood to lymph node.

of lymphocytes to where an antigen actually is, for example, the site of an infection. This latter process is mediated by various adhesion molecules on both lymphocytes and blood vessels and by special cytokines known as *chemokines*, as shown in Table 15.3. Note that T and B lymphocytes are not identical in their homing characteristics, and also that the recirculation of lymphocytes is quite distinct from that of cells of the myeloid lineage. Neutrophils circulate only through the bloodstream and do not enter the tissues except at local sites of inflammation or infection. Monocytes show an intermediate pattern, with a high baseline rate of entry into the tissues (up to 50% of blood monocytes per day) which is further increased in response to inflammation.

Antigen recognition molecules

As already mentioned, it is in recognition that lymphocytes excel. The surface molecules used by B and T cells are not the same, but they share one absolutely vital feature. They are put together from a combination of several genes in such a way that each lymphocyte carries a different combination and, as a result, recognizes a different antigen—or, in immunological jargon, displays a different

Table 15.3 Adhesion molecules involved in leucocyte migration, adhesion, and activation

Molecule/expressed on	Target cell	Effect
I. *Selectins*		
L selectin/leucocytes	HEV, endo	bind carbohydrates
P selectin/platelets; act endo	platelets, endo PMN	initial binding
E selectin/act endo	leucocytes	lymphocyte recirculation
II. *Integrins*		
LFA1/leucocyte subsets	endo, APC	adhesion and arrest
MAC-1 (CR3)/mono;	endo	leucocyte extravasation
PMN; mac	C3b on pathogens	via HEV or inflammation
VLA-1/PMN; T; mono.	endo	T cell–APC interactions
LPAM-1/lymphocytes;	endo	phagocytosis
mono		homing to gut
III. *Immunoglobulin superfamily*		
ICAM-1/DC; act endo	T cells; phagocytes	ligands for integrins
VCAM-1/act endo	PMN; T; mono	leucocyte migration
ICAM-3/naïve T cells	DC	T cell–APC interaction
Other		
CD44/memory T cells	endo/extracellular matrix	adhesion

endo: endothelium; act: activated; HEV: high endothelial venule; APC: antigen-presenting cell; DC: dendritic cell: mac: Macrophage; mono: monocyte; PMN: polymorphonuclear leucocyte; LFA: lymphocyte function antigen; ICAM: intercellular adhesion molecule.

specificity. The basic plan is shown in Fig. 15.3, and further details will be given in later chapters.

Clonal selection and memory

An individual lymphocyte that recognizes selectively 'its own' antigen (plus various signals from cytokines) will respond by proliferating into a population of lymphocytes with identical specificity. This population is referred to as a clone, and the sequence of (1) selection of one lymphocyte to respond and (2) expansion into a clone is known as *clonal selection*. The enlargement of lymph nodes during infection reflects the trapping of antigen-specific lymphocytes and their clonal expansion. Some of the members of the clone will then differentiate and carry out their function (the actual functions of B and T cells are different, see Chapters 16–19) while others stay behind as *memory cells*. Thus any subsequent (secondary) response to the same antigen will start from a larger number of lymphocytes of the right specificity, and the response will be faster and bigger, with

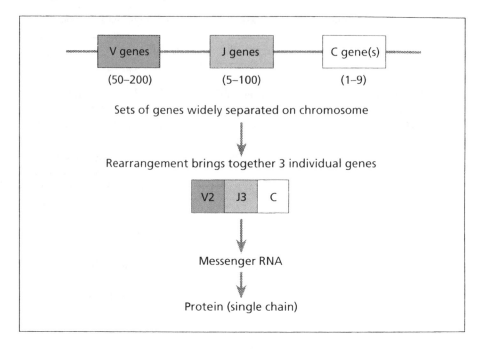

Fig. 15.3 The basic pattern of lymphocyte receptor generation. V, variable genes; J, joining genes; C, constant genes. In some cases there are also one or more D (diversity) genes between V and J. Since both the B cell receptor (antibody) and the T cell receptor are made up of two different chains, the possible combinations (the B and T cell 'repertoires') run into millions. This process of rearrangement occurs only in lymphocytes. In all other cells the genes remain in their original separated (and therefore non-functional) locations.

changes in antibody affinity (B cells) and triggering requirements (T cells) (Fig. 15.4). The host is now said to display memory for that particular antigen, and if the antigen is potentially dangerous—a bacterial toxin, for example—the difference between a secondary and a primary response may be the difference between life and death.

Regulation of adaptive immunity

Given this ability to proliferate and accelerate their response, lymphocytes clearly need fairly tight regulation, otherwise a single response would be in danger of occupying the entire system. In fact both B and T cells are under several types of control, involving both the death of cells and the inhibition of their proliferation (see Chapter 20 for further details), with the result that responses usually die down when they have achieved their purpose of eliminating the infection. But if elimination fails or regulation is faulty, *immunopathology* and *autoimmunity* may result, as you will see in Chapters 22 and 23.

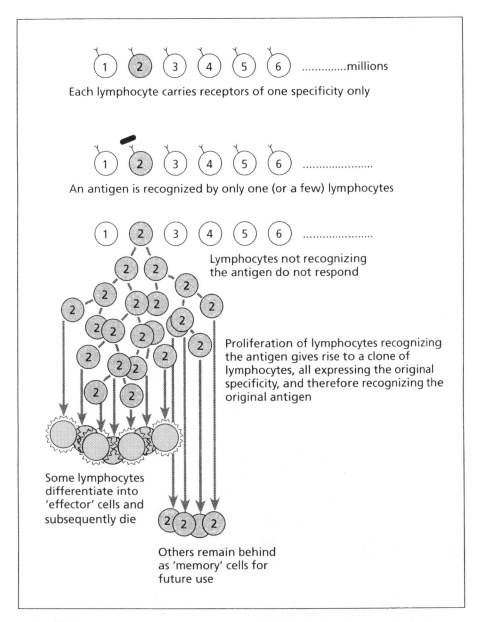

Each lymphocyte carries receptors of one specificity only

An antigen is recognized by only one (or a few) lymphocytes

Lymphocytes not recognizing the antigen do not respond

Proliferation of lymphocytes recognizing the antigen gives rise to a clone of lymphocytes, all expressing the original specificity, and therefore recognizing the original antigen

Some lymphocytes differentiate into 'effector' cells and subsequently die

Others remain behind as 'memory' cells for future use

Fig. 15.4 Adaptive immunity operates on the principle of clonal selection. Since individual lymphocytes rearrange their receptor genes differently (see Fig. 15.3), they express only one of the millions of possible specificities in the 'repertoire'. A lymphocyte recognizing a particular antigen is *selected* for expansion into a *clone* large enough to mount an effective response. Both B and T lymphocytes undergo clonal selection, though with slight differences in the later stages.

16 B cells and antibody

B lymphocytes (or 'B cells') are essentially little antibody factories, able to switch on high-rate synthesis and secretion of antibody molecules when stimulated by recognition of the 'right' antigen (the word *antigen* strictly implies a molecule that stimulates antibody production, but it is loosely used for any molecule recognized by a lymphocyte). When this happens the cell changes its appearance from the rather dull-looking lymphocyte, which is almost all nucleus, to the large plasma cell, with its cytoplasm full of rough endoplasmic reticulum (Fig. 16.1). High-rate antibody synthesis (up to 100 000 molecules per minute) can be kept up for 4–5 days, after which the plasma cell normally dies.

Recognition and response in B cells are perfectly coordinated, because their surface antigen-receptor is the *same molecule* (antibody) as they will secrete when stimulated. Thus only those antibody molecules are made that can bind to the stimulating antigen and help in its disposal, and production of unwanted antibodies is avoided. Having said this, it must be added that recognition is a relative matter (see below) and some of the antibody made during an infection probably binds too weakly—or in immunological jargon, is of too low *affinity*—to be of great use. However, the affinity of some antibodies is very high indeed, up to 10^{-11} molar, which is above the range of most enzyme–substrate interactions, and when thousands of antibody molecules bind to the surface of a virus or a bacteria, the microbe is doomed unless it takes evasive action (which many do, see Chapter 21). The diversity of the antibody repertoire is so enormous (look back to Chapter 15 to be reminded of the genetic recombination events that allow this) that it is very rare to find a microbial molecule, or even a totally synthetic one, against which antibody cannot be made.

The antibody molecule

Antibodies are globular proteins, whence the alternative name *immunoglobulins*. They are found predominantly in the gamma region on electrophoresis (but also in the beta and alpha 2 regions), and the name *gammaglobulin* is sometimes applied to crudely purified antibody preparations, for example, as used in treatment of antibody-deficient patients (see Chapters 24 and 27).

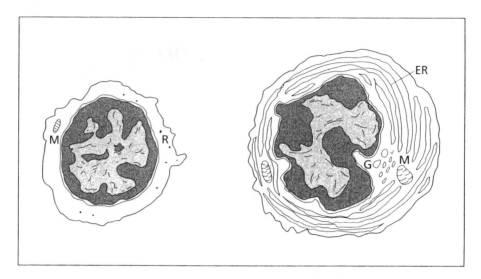

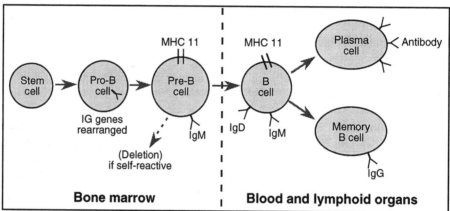

Fig. 16.1 *Top,* The resting B lymphocyte (*left*) has a small amount of cytoplasm, containing few organelles and only occasional ribosomes (R). The plasma cell (*right*) has more cytoplasm, mainly occupied by ribosome-rich rough endoplasmic reticulum (ER) which, together with the Golgi apparatus (G) is the site of high-rate antibody synthesis. M, mitochondria, more prominent in the metabolically active plasma cell. (× 8000). *Bottom,* B cells are produced by a series of maturation steps from precursors in the bone marrow.

Antibodies are made up of four polypeptide chains: two long or *heavy* chains and two short or *light* chains. The two heavy chains are identical and so are the two light chains, and each chain is coded for by genes rearranged as described in the previous chapter (see Fig. 15.3). The result is a Y-shaped molecule with the variable regions at the two tips of the Y and as its stem the constant region, to which only heavy chains, with their larger constant portions, contribute (Fig. 16.2). Even the constant regions of all antibody molecules are not identical, because there are nine different C genes and an individual B cell can use one or other of these, often switching C genes in mid-response. This is because different

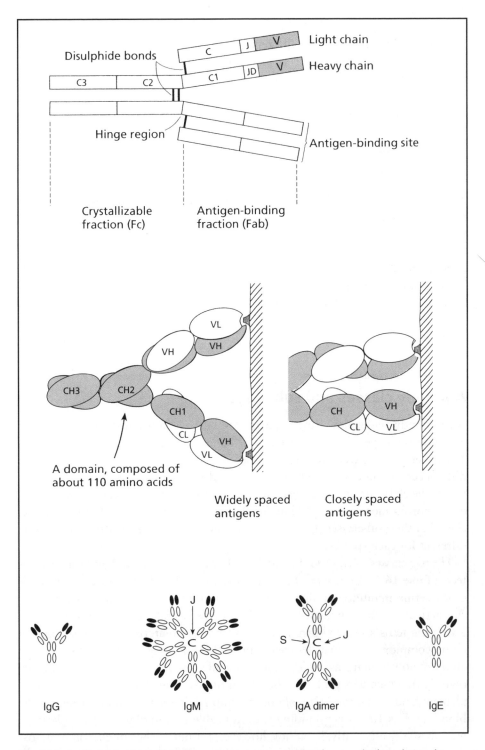

Fig. 16.2 Antibody structure. *Top*, diagrammatic representation, showing the four chains, the products of the rearranged genes, and some of the terminology. *Center*, how the molecule folds, emphasizing the repeating 'domain' structure and the value of the hinge region in adapting to differently spaced antigens. Both illustrations are of the IgG molecule. *Bottom*, the other classes differ in the number of C regions and disulphide bonds, and the total number of chains (Table 16.1). J: joining chain; S: secretary piece; dark: variable domains; light: constant domains.

constant regions can mediate different biological effects, including activation of innate immune elements such as phagocytic cells or complement (see below). Thus the antibody molecule can be seen as a focusing device linking the individual antigen, bound to one end, to a variety of disposal mechanisms to which the other end binds. In effect, the antibody is marking the antigen for disposal by the innate immune system.

Note that there are many other soluble molecules with the ability to bind to and dispose of pathogens, notably the collectins (see Chapter 11), but that none of these display the enormous discriminating power of antibody since their genes are not subject to recombination. A further interesting point about the antibody molecule is that its general structure—that is, the sequence of *domains* containing approximately 110 amino acids, and indeed some of the actual amino acid sequences themselves—is shared with a wide range of other molecules with connections to the immune system. Examples are the T-cell receptor and the MHC molecules (see Chapter 17) and various molecules involved in adhesion, lymphocyte activation, and binding antibody to cells which, together with antibody, are referred to as the *immunoglobulin superfamily*.

Antibody classes and subclasses

All antibody molecules using a particular heavy chain constant region gene, whatever their specificity for antigen, are defined as belonging to the same *class*. The differences between different classes are fairly major, but there are smaller differences within classes, which are referred to as *subclasses*. In evolutionary terms, the class differences go back to the earliest vertebrates, whereas subclasses have evolved more recently. Thus fishes, birds, and mammals all have the IgG class, but their subclasses (IgG1, IgG2, etc.) evolved independently and are quite different for each species.

The five classes—M, D, G, E, and A—differ considerably in their biological effects (Table 16.1). In general, IgG is the most useful and constitutes about 75% of the serum immunoglobulins. It is active both in the blood and in the tissues, can activate both complement and phagocytosis, and can cross the placenta, giving the fetus and newborn a protective level of maternal antibodies against many common infections. However, its half-life is only a few weeks, so after about 6 months maternal IgG is essentially all gone and the baby must make its own. IgM, which was probably the first antibody to evolve, also activates complement, and owing to its size (almost a million daltons, the largest protein in the blood) and its 10 antigen-binding sites, it is able to immobilize and agglutinate microbes very efficiently. It cannot, however, get out of the circulation or across the placenta. In its monomeric form it serves as the receptor molecule on B cells though after they have switched to IgG production (see Chapter 18) it is replaced

Table 16.1 Antibodies are divided into classes and subclasses according to the C genes used for their heavy chains. Here the essential characteristics and properties are shown for human antibodies. Note that activities not involving the Fc region (such as neutralization of toxins) can be performed by all classes of antibody

Class and subclass	Number of C domains	Molecular weight	Level in serum	Principal biological activities
IgM	4 (×5) (pentameric structure)	970 000	1.5 mg ml^{-1}	Agglutination Complement activation
IgD	3	184 000	30 µg ml^{-1}	B cell triggering
IgG1	3	146 000	9 mg ml^{-1}	Complement activation Opsonization for phagocytosis Reaches extravascular spaces Transfer across placenta
IgG2	3	146 000	3 mg ml^{-1}	As IgG1 but less
IgG3	3	170 000	1 mg ml^{-1}	As IgG1
IgG4	3	146 000	0.5 mg ml^{-1}	As IgG1, but does not activate complement
IgE basophils	4	188 000	50 ng ml^{-1}	Binds to mast cells and involved in allergies
IgA1 and 2 Serum	3	160 000	3.5 mg ml^{-1}	
Secretory (dimeric structure)	3 (×2)	380 000	—	Active in secretions

by IgG. This ability to *switch* classes without changing specificity—that is, to change Fc while retaining Fab—is another valuable consequence of the multi-gene arrangement of the Ig locus, and will be discussed further when we look at the antibody response (Chapter 18).

IgA is specially adapted to function at mucosal surfaces such as those in the intestine, lungs, urogenital system, and breast, and has additional components to protect it from proteolysis, which are acquired during its secretion into these sites. IgA accounts for about two-thirds of all Ig present in the body. IgE, present in only trace amounts, comes into prominence as the cause of allergies (see Chapter 21), but it is probably useful in setting off inflammatory responses; some believe its main function is in worm infections. IgD is found mainly on B cells rather than in serum, and is part of their activation pathway.

In addition to these heavy chain variants, there are two completely separate types of *light chain*, named lambda (λ) and kappa (κ), each with its own V, J, and C genes. A given antibody molecule has either both λ or both κ light chains (if it had one of each, the antigen-recognizing sites at the two ends of the Y would be different!). This choice of light chains doubles the already enormous number of possible antibody specificities. Yet another genetic variation is seen in the *allotypes*, which are small inherited differences, mainly in the C regions of the Ig molecule, somewhat analogous to the blood groups on red cells; like blood groups, their influence seems relatively minor but they can serve as useful genetic markers.

The antigen-binding site and antigenic determinants

What exactly do antibodies recognize? As Fig. 16.2 implies, only a very small part of the V domains is actually involved in binding the antigen—about 15–20 amino acids in fact, representing the tips of six *hypervariable* loops, three from the light chain and three from the heavy chain, coded for by those regions of the V gene where sequence variability is at its highest. Since these determine what shapes on the antigen the antibody will bind to, they are referred to as *complementarity determining regions* (CDR). The two domains fold in such a way that these six loops form a shallow patch or cavity about $700Å^2$ in size, large enough to make contact with, for example, 15–20 amino acids from a protein or six sugar residues from a polysaccharide (Fig. 16.3). The closer the molecules can approach, the tighter the fit (see *affinity*, below). Since this small portion of the antigen may be a unique shape, it follows that the binding site that fits it is also a unique shape, possibly found on only antibody molecules from that particular clone of B cells. This unique region of the antibody molecule is called the *idiotype* and has fascinating properties—for instance it can itself stimulate and bind to another antibody with a binding site complementary to it, which would then resemble the original antigen! This ability to mimic an antigen using an idiotype has found applications in experimental vaccination (see Chapter 27).

Thus we see that antibodies recognize three-dimensional shape, but not the shape of a whole bacterium or even virus, rather the shape of just a small portion of one of its surface molecules (also known as an antigenic *determinant* or *epitope*). Thus even the smallest virus can be recognized by a large number of different antibodies—as it were, 'looking at it' from different directions and 'seeing' different determinants. One slightly surprising consequence of the smallness of the antigenic site is that similar shapes occasionally occur by chance on completely different microbial or animal cells, so that an individual antibody stimulated by, for example, a bacterium, may be found to 'cross-react' with a completely unrelated microbe or even the cells of some foreign species of animal. Since microbial and animal cells are made up of essentially the same amino acids, sugars, etc., such cross-reactions are in fact quite common, and this may account for the unfortunate production of antibodies against 'self' molecules which occurs in some *autoimmune* diseases (see Chapter 23).

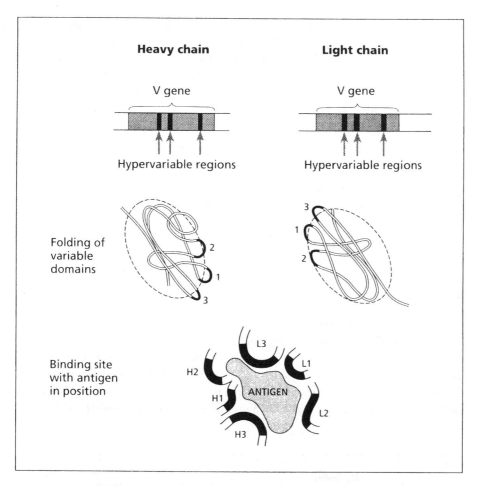

Fig. 16.3 The antigen-binding site, showing the location of the hypervariable regions in the V genes (*top*), their position in the folded variable immunoglobulin domain (*centre*), and how they make up the binding site (*bottom*, seen from 'end on' as the antigen molecule sees it). Note that the amino-acid sequences that make up the binding site are discontinuous; the same may be true of the amino acids or sugars making up the antigenic site.

Antibody affinity

As already mentioned, the affinity of the antibody–antigen bond can be very high, ranging from 10^{-7} to 10^{-11} molar. Nevertheless, it must be stressed that it is a non-covalent bond, capable of coming apart, the affinity being merely the expression of this probability. The forces that hold antibody and antigen together are the usual intermolecular ones—hydrophobic, hydrogen bonding, electrostatic, and van der Waals. During the antibody response (see Chapter 18) the average affinity of all the antibody in the serum rises, owing partly to selection of the highest affinity B cells and partly to small random improvements in the antibody-combining site by mutation, so that antibody formed later in the response, and in subsequent responses, is even better adapted to the antigen in question. These unusually frequent mutations in the CDR genes of individual B cells, inherited by the progeny of that cell, are an example of *somatic hypermutation*. Note that the term *affinity* applies to the binding of one antibody-combining site–antigen bond; in practice, since antibodies are at least divalent it is the total strength or *avidity* that matters.

What antibodies do

Antibody functions in three main ways: on its own to *neutralize* threatening molecules or pathogens; in conjunction; with cells to promote *phagocytosis*; and to activate the powerful effects of *complement* (see Fig. 16.4).

Neutralization

One of the first properties of antibody to be discovered was its ability to neutralize bacterial toxins, such as those of tetanus, diphtheria, etc., which forms the basis of vaccines against these diseases, and of the ability of injected antibody to save life in an acute infection ('passive immunization'). This is simply a matter of the Ig molecule blocking the binding of the toxin to the cell receptor via which it enters and damages cells. A similar process can effectively prevent the entry of

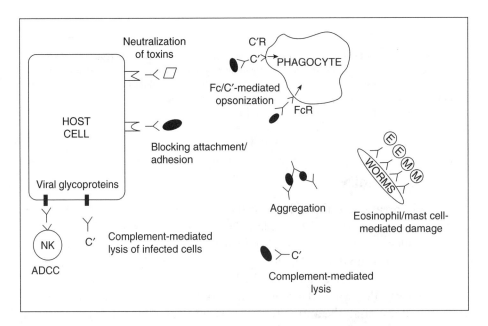

Fig. 16.4 A summary of the protective effects of antibody.

Table 16.2 Summary of Fc and complement receptors

Receptor	Expressed by (*induced)	Binds to	Effect on cell function
FcγRI (CD64)	Macrophages, dendritic cells neutrophils*, eosinophils*	IgG1 = IgG3 >G4 > G2	Uptake, activation, respiratory burst/ microbicidal activity, antigen presentation
FcγRII A (CD32)	Macrophages, neutrophils, eosinophils, Langerhans cells, platelets	IgG1 > G3 = G2 > G4	Uptake, eosinophil degranulation
FcγRII B1 (CD32)	B cells, mast cells	IgG1 = G3 > G4 > G2	No uptake, inhibition
FcγRII B2 (CD32)	Macrophages, neutrophils, eosinophils	IgG1 = G3 > G4 > G2	Uptake, inhibition
FcγRIII A (CD16)	NK cells	IgG1 = G3	Killing, cytokine secretion
FcγRIII B (CD16)	Eosinophils, macrophages, neutrophils, mast cells	IgG1 = G3	Uptake, activation
FcεRI	Mast cells, basophils, eosinophils*	IgE (high affinity)	Degranulation
FcεRII (CD23)	B cells, macrophages, eosinophils	IgE (low affinity)	Activation
FcαRI (CD89)	Monocytes*, neutrophils*, eosinophils	IgA (low affinity)	Uptake, activation, respiratory burst, antigen presentation
CR1 (CD35)	Follicular dendritic cells, B cells, monocytes, macrophages, erythrocytes, neutrophils, eosinophils, some T cells	C3b, C4b	Binds immune complexes, phagocytosis (with C5a)
CR2 (CD21)	B cells, follicular dendritic cells, some T cells	C3d, C3dg, iC3b	Binds EBV, B cell activation (component of B cell receptor complex)
CR3 (CD11b/18)	Monocytes, macrophages, neutrophils, NK cells, some T cells	iC3b	Phagocytosis, cell adhesion
CR4 (CD11c/18)	As above	iC3b	As above
C3a/4aR	Mast cells, basophils	C3a, 4a	Degranulation
C5aR	Mast cells, basophils, monocytes, macrophages, neutrophils, platelets, endothelial cells	C5a	Degranulation, migration, and adhesion of phagocytes to endothelium

viruses into their intended target cells and is the basis for many, though not all, virus vaccines (see Chapters 27 and 30).

Phagocytosis

In Chapter 11 we described how phagocytic cells such as macrophages and polymorphs can bind to many pathogens through 'pattern-recognition' of their surface features. The presence of antibody bound to the pathogen extends this recognition to potentially *any* pathogen, because now the cell can recognize the antibody molecule itself by virtue of the presence of 'Fc receptors' into which the end of the molecule opposite to that binding the pathogen can dock (see Fig. 16.2 and Table 16.2).

Complement

Chapter 11 also describes how antibody bound to an antigen can activate the classical complement pathway, leading to even more potent phagocytosis, because phagocytes possess receptors for the cleavage fragment C3b (see Table 16.2), as well as to the promotion of inflammation and, in some cases, lysis of the pathogen.

Thus members of the triad antibody + complement + phagocytes frequently operate together, especially in dealing with bacteria, and the main effects of a deficiency of any one of the triad are much the same—an increased incidence of bacterial infection. The added power contributed by antibody is illustrated by the inability of innate immunity (i.e. complement + phagocytes) to control many infections until sufficient antibody has been made, one of the best examples being streptococcal ('pneumococcal') pneumonia, where the patient is desperately ill until about a week after infection—the time it takes for a significant amount of IgG to be made (see Chapter 12).

The antibody industry

Another useful role of antibody (not anticipated by Nature!) is as a *targeting* device for toxic drugs, radioactive molecules, etc. in the monitoring and treatment of disease. Antibodies are also invaluable in the laboratory for *typing* cells (e.g. red cells for blood transfusion) because they can identify the small differences carried on the molecules of different blood groups, and for identifying pathogens in *diagnosis*. For such purposes the purer the antibody the better, and as a result of steady technical improvements, the production of pure antibody has progressed to the point where virtually unlimited amounts of antibody of any specificity can be synthesized. So important was the invention of *monoclonal antibody* technology that it earned the Nobel Prize for Köhler and Milstein.

17 T cells and the MHC

Resting T lymphocytes look very much like resting B lymphocytes, but when they respond the difference becomes apparent: instead of turning into plasma cells and secreting antibody, they enlarge slightly and secrete *cytokines* and/or *toxic molecules* with effects on other cells, but with no specificity towards particular antigens. As the effects of these molecules are usually fairly short range, it is the cell to which the T cell responds (the 'target' cell) that receives the main impact, so that T cell responses essentially operate at close quarters. Depending on the type of T lymphocyte, this effect can result in the target cell being activated or killed (Table 17.1), the common feature being that the T cell is responding to changes detected on the surface of the target cell but reflecting the presence of foreign material *inside* it—the 'internal environment'. In a typical situation such as a virus infection, the T cell makes use of the ability of target cells to convey small bits of viral protein (i.e. peptides) from inside the cell to the cell surface, using a special set of molecules known as MHC proteins (for *major histocompatibility complex*; see later for an explanation of this strange name). Since these peptides are derived from a foreign microbe (in this case a virus) there will be, among the repertoire of T cells, a few whose receptors recognize that combination of MHC and peptide and only these T cells will respond. Thus although the effects of T cells are non-specific, their recognition of antigen is highly specific. But T cells do not only recognize protein fragments; glycolipid antigens are recognized too, though here another set of antigen-presenting molecules known as CD1 are involved, as will be explained later.

Subpopulations of T cells

Not all T cells have the same range of functions (see Table 17.1). The major distinction is between *cytotoxic* and *helper* (or strictly speaking, *cytokine secreting*) cells. Cytotoxic T cells are predominantly equipped to kill cells harbouring intracellular pathogens such as viruses, while helper cells are designed to switch on or enhance the activity of B lymphocytes, macrophages, and other cells involved in defence, as described in the following two chapters. The process by which antigens reach the surface of these cells is described below. Obviously it is vital

Table 17.1 The main types of T lymphocytes and their functions.

Common name	Receptor chains	Characteristic surface marker	Main secreted product	Cells affected	Main effect
Cytotoxic (CTL)	α/β	CD8	Perforins, 'granzymes' Cytokines (IFNγ)	Any nucleated cell	Killing (especially viruses)
Helper (T_H1)	α/β	CD4	Cytokines (especially IFNγ)	Macrophages	Activation
(T_H2)	α/β	CD4	Cytokines (especially IL- 4,5,13)	B lymphocytes	Proliferation Antibody secretion
Regulatory	α/β	CD4	IL-10, TGFβ	T, B lymphocytes Macrophages	Inhibition
Gamma/ delta	γ/δ		IFNγ	Macrophages	Activation Regulation

CD: cluster of differentiation, a terminology used for cell-surface molecules, of which at least 160 are now recognized.

for these two quite different effects to be applied to the right target cell and this is ensured by another set of surface molecules on the T cells. One, known as CD4, is found mainly on helper T cells, and recognizes one set of MHC molecules (class II, see below); thus helper T cells will only help cells bearing MHC class II, which normally means B cells, macrophages, and dendritic cells. Another, known as CD8, is found mainly on cytotoxic cells, and recognizes MHC class I molecules, which are carried by all nucleated cells (i.e. all but red blood cells). The biological sense is excellent, because only B cells, macrophages, and dendritic cells can benefit from 'help', whereas any cell may pick up a virus and will then need to be killed. Figure 17.1 illustrates these interactions and the processes are described further in Chapter 19. There are also T cells whose main function appears to be to *regulate* other cells, sometimes switching them off—a process vital to all adaptive immune responses (see Chapter 20).

What T cells recognize

Proteins

One cannot discuss the T cell receptor without also discussing MHC molecules, since they usually act together in protein recognition; that is, the most commonly expressed T cell receptor (α/β) will not respond to a peptide unless it is bound to

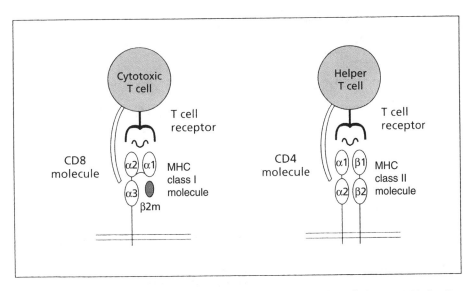

Fig. 17.1 Interactions between T cells and MHC molecules. The binding of CD8 to MHC class I, and of CD4 to class II, ensures that cytotoxic and helper T cells only interact with an appropriate target cell. ~ represents a peptide antigen.

an MHC molecule. This again makes excellent biological sense because MHC molecules are found on cell surfaces and T cells can only do something useful to a cell; their secreted products in the majority of cases cannot affect microbes directly. Thus the presence of MHC molecules advertises the presence of a *cell*, and the presence of a foreign peptide bound to it advertises the presence of a *foreign* microbe inside the cell: an ingenious way for one cell to 'look inside' another!

T cell receptors are so heterogeneous that an individual T cell will preferentially recognize one unique combination of MHC molecule and microbial peptide, although this restriction is not absolute (see Chapter 23). The peptide, lying in the long narrow binding cleft on the MHC molecule, will no longer be in the three-dimensional form in which it occurred in the larger protein it was derived from. So the T cell receptor recognizes *continuous linear* protein fragments, unlike antibody which recognizes three-dimensional shapes that may be discontinuous parts of protein or sugar (look back to Fig. 16.3). And since it only recognizes a peptide bound to the right MHC molecule, such a response is referred to as 'MHC restricted'. Figure 17.2 illustrates these basic principles.

Interestingly, MHC restriction is involved in T cell development even before any contact with foreign antigens, because in the thymus, where T cells mature, they are exposed to the combination of self-MHC and self-peptides in a complex process that ensures that the minimum of self-reactive T cells and the maximum of foreign-reactive ones reach the peripheral lymphoid organs. These events are referred to as *negative* and *positive* selection, respectively.

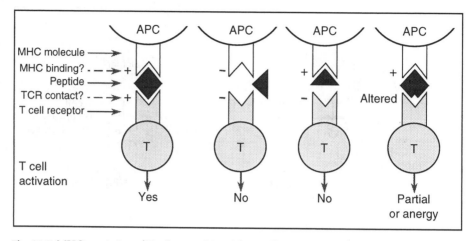

Fig. 17.2 MHC restriction of T cell recognition. The T cell shown here recognizes only one combination of MHC and bound peptide. Other T cells will recognize other combinations. Note that a given peptide may bind to several (though not all) MHC molecules. T cell activation will not occur if the peptide fails to bind both MHC and T cell receptor. Subtle modifications in amino acids of otherwise immunogenic peptides (so called altered peptide ligands) may lead to partial T cell activation or anergy.

Glycolipids and carbohydrates

To present non-protein molecules a completely different set of presenting structures is used, the CD1 molecules which bind lipid-containing molecules via their hydrophobic lipid portions (see below and Table 17.2). There is apparently no specialized molecule for presenting a pure carbohydrate, as mentioned in Chapter 18, many carbohydrates do not *require* T cells in order to induce antibody.

Antigen-presenting molecules

The MHC and its molecules

At this point, a digression is required to explain the MHC in more detail. As mentioned above, the initials stand for Major Histocompatibility Complex, which is the name given to a large genetic region containing the genes that determine the success or failure of graft rejection. If two individuals have the same set of MHC molecules (as identical twins do) they will not reject each other's grafts; if they differ (as unrelated people do) there will be some degree of rejection. Although this is historically the way in which the MHC was discovered, it is, of course, not the real function of the MHC, which as stated above is to transport

Table 17.2 MHC and CD1 molecules compared

	MHC class I	MHC class II	CD1 group 1	CD1 group 2
Genes	HLA A,B,C	HLA DP, DQ, DR	CD1a,b,c	CD1d
Chains	α, β2M	α, β	α, β2M	α, β2M
Polymorphism	++	++	–	–
Ligands	Peptides (8–11aa)	Peptides (10–30aa)	(Glyco)lipids e.g. mycobacteria	(Glyco)lipids α-galactosyl ceramide, parasite GPI?
Antigen Processing	+	+	(+)	?
Expressed on	All nucleated cells	DC, mac, B cells	DC, B cells	Mono, mac, etc.
Responding cells	CD8+ T (TcR α/β)	CD4+ T (TcR α/β)	CD4-/8- T, CD8+ T (TcR α/β, γ/δ)	NKT (TcR α/β restricted)

Key: aa: amino acids; TcR: T cell receptor; DC: dendritic cell; mono: monocyte; mac: macrophage; GPI: glycosyl phosphatidylinositol.

and 'present' foreign peptides to T cells. The MHC is extraordinarily polymorphic, some loci having up to 150 allelic variants, and as they are heterodimers (made up of two different chains) there are an estimated 10^{13} different possible combinations, so that identity between two individuals (other than identical twins) is virtually impossible.

There is no obvious reason why everybody's MHC antigens should differ in this way, but it is generally assumed to be something to do with ensuring that everybody does not respond identically to every infection; if they did, the argument goes, a new one might wipe out the entire species. Be that as it may, differences in MHC type are undoubtedly responsible for some of the differences in the responses of individuals to the same infection (see Chapter 26 for a further discussion of this point). Evolutionists speculate that the MHC and the T cell receptor developed together, in invertebrate days, as a recognition pair involved in normal cell adhesion. Interestingly, both of them, together with antibody and many other molecules, share enough DNA homology, including the all-important *domain* pattern, to suggest that they originated from the same primordial gene, and they are collectively known as the *immunoglobulin superfamily*.

Human MHC molecules (in man, the MHC is referred to as HLA, for 'human leucocyte antigen') are of two types, known as class I and class II, with slightly different structure and function (Fig. 17.3). There are three kinds of class I

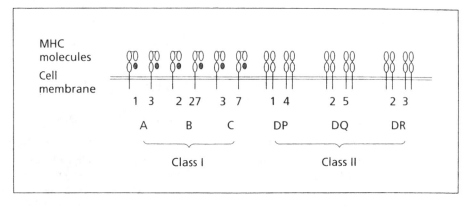

Fig. 17.3 MHC (HLA) genes and the corresponding molecules in the membrane of a human cell. Because there are many alleles at each locus, the number of combinations is astronomical (about 10^{13}). The cells of this individual would be typed as A 1,3; B 2,27; C 3,7; DP 1,4; DQ 2,5; DR 2,3. The small black circles represent β2 microglobulin, a quite separate molecule that stabilizes class I molecules.

molecule (A, B, and C) and three of class II (DP, DQ, and DR). Since they are *co-dominantly* expressed (i.e. both parental chromosomes are used), each cell carries two sets of molecules of each kind, twelve in all. Class I molecules are found on all nucleated cells, class II only on some; this is part of the process of selecting the right type of T cell for the job (e.g. killing or help). The MHC is a large locus, and the class I and II genes are separated by a number of other genes of immunological interest, including those for several cytokines and complement components as well as for the proteasomes and transporter proteins used for antigen processing (see below).

CD1 molecules

These are not part of the MHC, but they do have some structural resemblance to MHC Class I molecules and like them are associated with a smaller molecule called *β2 microglobulin*. However they lack the enormous polymorphism of MHC molecules, there being just four types: CD1 a,b,c (group 1), and d (group 2). As Table 17.2 shows, Group 1 CD molecules follow trafficking pathways within the antigen-presenting cell enabling them to pick up glycolipids from either endogenous or exogenous pathogens for presentation to T cells (see *antigen processing*, below) while those of group 2 are specialized for presenting to NKT cells. As one might predict, the best-established microbial ligands for group 1 molecules are glycolipids from mycobacteria—intracellular organisms renowned for their almost impenetrable waxy cell wall—the lipid portion being held in the CD1 binding groove and the hydrophilic sugar residues presented to the T cell receptor (Fig. 17.2). The apparently unique ligand for group 2 is α-galactosyl ceramide, a glycolipid originally derived from sea sponges and not yet identified on microbes.

Table 17.3 T and B cell receptors compared

	T cell receptor	Antibody molecule
Recombination of V–J–C genes	In T cells only	In B cells only
Junctional diversity	Yes	Yes
Subsequent mutation	No	Yes
Chains	α and β, or γ and δ	2 heavy (M, G, D, A, or E) and 2 light (κ or λ)
Molecular weight	95 000	146 000–970 000
Recognizes	(1) Small linear peptides (9–15 amino acids) plus MHC molecule (2) Glycolipids plus CD1 molecules	Three-dimensional shape of proteins and sugars
Secreted into blood	No	Yes

The T cell receptor

The antigen receptor on the T cell has similarities to the antibody molecule, but with important differences (Table 17.3). Unlike the antibody on the B cell, which can be thought of as a sample of what that cell can produce, like the goods in a shop window, the T cell receptor can be thought of rather like a hand reaching out to feel the surface of neighbouring cells, with some fingers devoted to contacting MHC molecules and others probing for the peptide bound to them (Fig. 17.1).

Antigen processing and presentation

Processing

An intracellular virus or other pathogen is, in immunological terms, a large complex structure, and to convert it into a series of small peptides in the groove of the MHC molecules on the cell surface, quite complicated processes must occur. These take place in the *antigen-presenting cells* (APC), which may be dendritic cells, macrophages, or B lymphocytes. A pathogen or its molecules can be intracellular for two reasons: (1) *exogenously*, i.e. actively taken into the presenting cell by phagocytosis, of which bacteria are typical examples, for presentation by MHC class II molecules to CD4 T cells; and (2) *endogenously*, i.e. already growing in the APC—particularly viruses—and presented via MHC class I

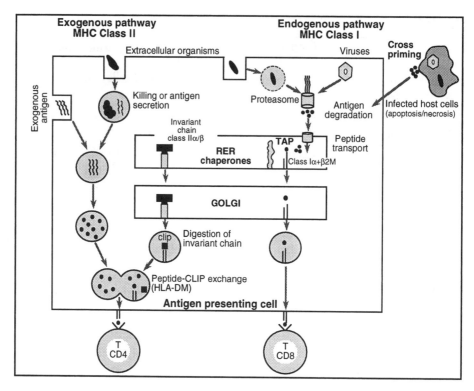

Fig. 17.4 Pathways of antigen processing. RER: rough endoplasmic reticulum; TAP: transporter associated with antigen processing.

molecules to CD8 T cells. Each type is handled by a different set of intracellular processes (Fig. 17.4).

The exogenous (class II) pathway

Like all phagocytosed material (see Chapter 11), an engulfed bacterium will normally end up in an endosome (phagolysosome) where it is digested at acid pH by proteases into short peptides of up to about 20 amino acids. These endosomes fuse with Golgi-derived vesicles containing MHC class II molecules whose groove is temporarily blocked by a molecule called invariant chain; this is now exchanged for the bacterial peptide. The new MHC–peptide complex is then transported to the cell surface to be recognized by CD4 T cells (see below). Not surprisingly, some successful pathogens can interfere with this process, for example by inhibiting endosomal proteases (e.g. the roundworm *Brugia*) or blocking phagosome–lysosome fusion (e.g. *M. tuberculosis*).

The endogenous (class I) pathway

Here it is a question of getting peptides newly synthesised in the cytoplasm of the host cell onto the cell membrane bound to MHC class I molecules. This involves specialized structures called *proteasomes* that chop proteins into peptides of rather precise length (8–10 amino acids) which just fit the MHC class I groove, and *transporter* proteins (TAP) that carry them across the membranes of the endoplasmic reticulum (ER). Here they meet MHC molecules in the course of assembly. Golgi vesicles then bud off from the ER and carry the MHC–peptide complex to the cell surface to be recognized by CD8 T cells. Note that neither pathway incorporates any mechanism for distinguishing foreign from 'self' proteins, and in fact even during a virus infection only a small proportion of MHC class I molecules will carry viral peptides, most of them being loaded with self peptides. Note also that the two pathways are not in practice quite so rigidly separate since, to give one example, an APC could acquire viral proteins by phagocytosing material from cells lysed by the virus, which would then proceed through the exogenous pathway to CD4 T cells. In practice most pathogens elicit both CD4 and CD8 responses to some degree.

Presentation and costimulation

It is not sufficient merely to display MHC–peptide complexes on the APC surface to activate T cells. Even when the T cell receptor binds to the peptide, several *costimulatory* non-antigen specific molecular interactions are also required. Two have already been mentioned: the binding of CD4 on the T cell to MHC class II on the APC, and the binding of CD8 to MHC class I; these ensure that the appropriate type of T cell is activated, e.g. CD4 helpers for a macrophage struggling to eliminate mycobacteria versus CD8 killers for a virally infected cell. Other essential interactions involve molecules induced on the APC by the pathogen itself (e.g. B7, which binds to CD28 on T cells); these help to ensure that T cells concentrate their attention on infected rather than normal cells and that the initial contact between T cell and APC proceeds to firmer, more prolonged binding and optimal activation (Fig. 17.5). Thus there are important quantitative and temporal elements to antigen presentation. To sum up this whole complex process, its outcome depends on (1) properties of the antigen: which proteases generate which peptides, (2) the available MHC molecules, since these have a broad but not infinite range of peptide-binding capacities, and (3) the repertoire of T cell receptors for the MHC–peptide complexes produced. The result is inevitably a hierarchy of antigens from each pathogen, some being more effective ('immunodominant') than others while some components of the pathogens may not function as antigens at all.

Superantigens

There is one exception to the normal 'MHC-restricted' pattern of T cell responses to proteins described above. Some microbial proteins, notably the

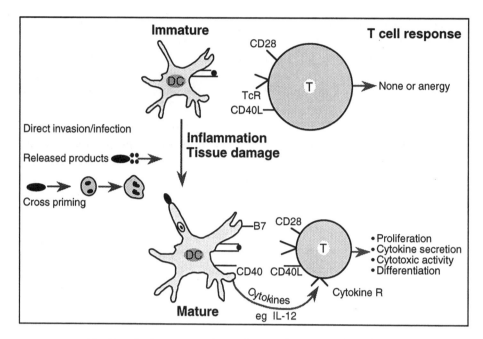

Fig. 17.5 Antigen presentation and costimulation. DC, dendritic cell.

enterotoxins of staphylococci, have the ability to stimulate a substantial number of T cells, for example up to 20%, instead of the one per million or so expected if the recognition were receptor specific. These responses do require class II MHC molecules, but are not restricted to a single MHC type. The explanation is thought to be that these 'superantigens' bind to parts of the MHC and the T cell receptor (always the same one of the two variable domains known as Vß), *outside* the usual polymorphic peptide binding site, though some may also interact with the peptide. The stimulation of so many T cells at once and the release of huge amounts of pro-inflammatory cytokines such as IL-2 and TNF α and β, together with IL-1 from activated macrophages, contributes to the toxicity of these antigens, which can be terrifying. For example, *Staphylococcus aureus* and *Streptococcus pyogenes*, which together have no less than 21 different superantigens, can cause massive fatal food poisoning and the toxic shock syndrome. There are also viral superantigens. Exactly what role these bizarre responses play, and even whether they are of use to the pathogen or the host, is still a mystery.

γδ T cells

Yet another exception to 'classical' presentation as described earlier is the γδ T cells, which constitute a minor (1–5%) fraction of all T cells but are enriched in the intestinal mucosal epithelium (Table 17.1). These can recognize phosphate-containing molecules (e.g. on mycobacteria) by a process involving their TCR but not MHC or CD1. Their role in infection is still somewhat mysterious; they can produce IFNγ and IL-10 and may play a role in limiting local tissue damage.

18 The antibody response

Lymphocytes do not just *function*; they *respond* by proliferating into clones, changing their size and shape, and secreting important molecules. As emphasized in Chapters 15–17, B and T lymphocytes differ in many respects, and this includes the way they respond. In this chapter we will consider how B cells and T cells, acting together, give rise to the production of antibody molecules—the *antibody response*.

The antibody response illustrates perfectly the principles of adaptive immunity. Consider the life-story of a typical individual with respect to *Streptococcus pneumoniae* (the pneumococcus) in the days before antibiotics. At birth, if the mother has previously had pneumonia, the baby will acquire some antibody specific for the bacterium across the placenta (see Chapter 16), so he or she is protected against infection. By about 6–9 months most of this is gone, and the baby is now susceptible to infection, though pneumonia with this organism is in fact commoner at older ages. If it does develop, the patient is severely ill for about a week, during which time innate immune mechanisms (mainly phagocytes and complement) struggle to control the rapidly growing organisms. But *antibody* production has begun, and after a week the IgG antibody in the blood reaches a level sufficient to opsonize all the bacteria, the *phagocytes* home in, and a few hours later the patient is miraculously better. This illustrates the time lag characteristic of primary antibody responses.

A second infection with the same strain of pneumococcus will be met by a secondary antibody response so rapid that the patient will be unaware of the infection. This illustrates *memory*. However, infection with a different strain (there are at least 80) will require production of a different antibody, because of the very high specificity of antibody for the antigens of the bacterium; meanwhile the patient will again develop serious pneumonia (Fig. 18.1). You can nowadays be *vaccinated* against this disease, but a complete vaccine would have to contain over 80 different antigens! (In practice, about 50 are enough to protect most people.) Patients who for some reason are *deficient* in producing antibody are extremely susceptible to this type of infection, but they can be kept healthy by monthly injections of immunoglobulin pooled from large numbers of normal people, showing that (1) it really is antibody that protects, and (2) normal people have protective levels of it.

For the production of a typical IgG antibody response such as that described

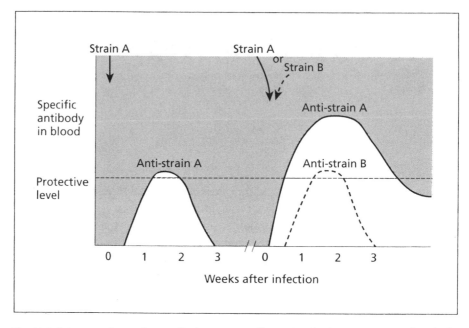

Fig. 18.1 Primary and secondary antibody responses, illustrating the slow appearance of antibody in the primary response, and the faster and greater response to a second contact with the same antigen. If the first contact with strain A had been in the form of a non-pathogenic vaccine, subsequent infection would lead directly to a secondary response. For details of the difference between primary and secondary antibody, see Table 18.2.

above, four events must take place: activation of B cells; presentation of antigen to T cells; activation of T cells; and 'help' for the B cells by T cells.

Activation of B cells

This occurs mainly in the lymphoid organs (lymph nodes, spleen, etc.). Different sorts of antigen activate B cells in different ways. Some do not in fact require T cell help, and are known as *T-independent* (Ti antigens). This may be because they have intrinsic *mitogenic* activity (Ti I antigens such as LPS)—that is, they induce mitosis, or cell division, in many B cells, followed by antibody secretion (Fig. 18.2(a)). Others (Ti II), consisting of *repeated identical antigenic determinants* can stimulate specific B cells to divide and secrete antibody, by binding to and linking together several of their surface immunoglobulin receptors (Fig. 18.2(b)). Ti II antigens include many of the polysaccharides in the capsules of dangerous bacteria such as the meningococcus, *Haemophilus*, and *S. pneumoniae*, and the antibody they induce, though it may be life-saving, lacks some of the features of the T-dependent responses described below, such as class switching, affinity maturation, and memory. Moreover, Ti II antigens tend to inactivate

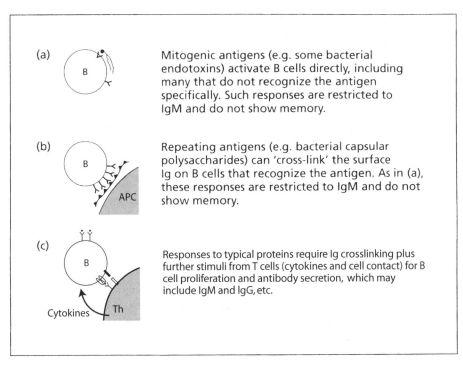

(a) Mitogenic antigens (e.g. some bacterial endotoxins) activate B cells directly, including many that do not recognize the antigen specifically. Such responses are restricted to IgM and do not show memory.

(b) Repeating antigens (e.g. bacterial capsular polysaccharides) can 'cross-link' the surface Ig on B cells that recognize the antigen. As in (a), these responses are restricted to IgM and do not show memory.

(c) Responses to typical proteins require Ig crosslinking plus further stimuli from T cells (cytokines and cell contact) for B cell proliferation and antibody secretion, which may include IgM and IgG, etc.

Fig. 18.2 B cells can be activated in three ways, corresponding to different types of antigen. Note that (a) and (b) illustrate 'T-cell-independent' responses and (c) illustrates a 'T-cell-dependent' response. B, B lymphocyte; Th, CD4 T helper cell.

rather than activate the B cells of very young children, who therefore do not mount good antibody responses to pathogens such as *Haemophilus influenzae* and *Neisseria meningitidis* unless they are combined with a protein carrier as they are in protein–polysaccharide–conjugate vaccines. Note that the original definition of a T-independent antigen was that it induced antibody in animals lacking thymuses and *most* T cells, as some bacterial polysaccharides can; however, this does not mean that some T cells cannot recognize and provide help for polysaccharides and some lipids, and in fact Ti II antigens can derive help from the Tγδ subpopulation of T cells (see Chapter 17).

Mitogenic and repeating antigens are relatively restricted and most pathogen-derived molecules, particularly proteins, have neither of these two properties; for them to activate B cells, several molecules need to be 'presented' to the B cell simultaneously, and this is done by special *antigen-presenting cells*, found mainly in the lymphoid organs (Fig. 18.2(c)). This type of response also requires further 'help' from T cells (see below), and for this reason it is referred to as 'T-dependent' (TD). The ability of protein antigens to enlist T help is made use of in the improvement of polysaccharide vaccines by conjugating them to proteins (see Chapter 27).

Activation through the B cell antigen receptor complex

The immunoglobulin molecule in the surface of the B cell, though it does penetrate the membrane, has no intrinsic enzymatic activity—so how does it switch on the intracellular mechanisms that lead to antibody formation? The answer is that it is associated in the membrane with other molecules that can transduce signals from outside the cell to the nucleus; these together form the B cell receptor complex (BCR). Without the BCR, a B cell cannot respond, and interestingly there are B-cell-infecting viruses, such as EBV and HHV8, which can inhibit BCR function, presumably to evade recognition and promote their own survival. Signal transduction via the BCR is not 'all or nothing'; it depends on the extent and duration of interaction and is influenced by such factors as antigen valency, state of aggregation, and persistence. In fact under certain conditions it can induce not responsiveness but unresponsiveness, and even death of the B cell! In addition to the BCR other *costimulatory* molecules play a part in B cell activation; these include CD19, CD81, CR2, and probably IgD. The involvement of CR2 (the receptor for the complement factor C3d) explains why depletion of C3, e.g. by cobra venom factor, inhibits antibody responses, and also why conjugation of C3d to an antigen makes it a more powerful inducer of antibody—a potentially useful adjunct to vaccination.

During normal activation by a multivalent antigen, clusters or 'arrays' of these BCR and costimulatory molecules are drawn together into so-called *lipid rafts*—areas of altered lipid composition floating in the plasma membrane phospholipid bilayer, which selectively promote molecular interactions and signal transduction. It is thought that the inhibitory effect of EBV mentioned above is partly due to blocking the formation of lipid rafts. This 'cross-linking' of the BCR in turn improves the ability of the B cell to present antigen to T cells by increasing the levels of costimulatory molecules (see below). When we consider the activation of T cells, you will see many similarities to B cell activation, particularly in the existence of costimulatory molecules, though there are differences too.

Consequences of activation: proliferation and differentiation

Whatever the route of activation, B cells need to proliferate into a large enough population to make the enormous numbers of antibody molecules required for a useful response. Note that in the examples shown in Fig. 18.2(b) and (c) this proliferation only occurs in antigen-specific B cells—i.e. it is *clonal*—whereas in Fig. 18.2(a) the proliferation would be *polyclonal* and much of the antibody would not react with the inducing antigen. This is because Ti I antigens do not act through the highly specific B cell receptor complex whereas Ti II and TD antigens do.

Proliferation involves entry into cell cycle and cell division; differentiation refers to enlargement of the cell and its organelles, with a visible change from lymphocyte to *plasma cell* morphology, and the increased expression of anti-apoptotic molecules that increase survival as well as molecules that facilitate interaction with T cells. Further differentiation steps include the switch from secreting IgM to IgG, IgA, etc. (see below) and the generation of memory cells (see Chapter 20).

Presentation of antigen to T cells

In Chapter 17 it was stressed that, though T cells can undoubtedly respond to some glycolipids, the responses to proteins are best understood. Here what the T cells actually recognize are *small peptides* bound to *MHC molecules*, so for them to be activated a presenting cell is needed, and it must display MHC molecules of the appropriate class, associated with a peptide derived from the interior of the cell. These presenting cells are of three types: antigen-specific B cells, macrophages, and specialized antigen-presenting *dendritic* cells. One of the functions of lymphoid organs is to facilitate close contact between B and T cells. In general, the dendritic cells are more important in primary responses, when there are relatively few B cells of the right specificity available; in secondary responses and at sites of infection, B cells and macrophages become major sources of antigen presentation.

Let us consider B cells first (Fig. 18.3, steps 1–5(b)). Following activation of a B cell as in Fig. 18.2(c), the complex of antigen plus BCR is taken into the cell, and the antigen is 'processed', i.e. digested by enzymes so that its constituent peptides can be picked up by the newly synthesised MHC class II molecules, which are then transported to the cell surface. This processing into peptides is not in itself restricted to foreign antigens, but is tremendously more efficient (up to a million times) with foreign antigens because of their association with the BCR, which is where the specificity lies. Any CD4-bearing T cell that recognizes this combination of MHC and peptide will be activated to proliferate into a clone of helper T cells capable of helping any B cell carrying the same combination of MHC+peptide. This means that B cells whose own Ig receptor binds one part of an antigen can be helped by T cells that recognize another part. Note that the B and T cells do not have to recognize the same portion of the antigen—indeed almost invariably they do not, and the terms *B epitope* and *T epitope* are used to describe parts of the antigen 'seen' by B and T cells, respectively. Historically this distinction was worked out using small chemical groups conjugated to proteins—*haptens* and *carriers*—a situation that can occur naturally, e.g. in allergic responses to penicillin. Normally the result is a beautifully integrated process by which only B cells of the right specificity receive help—though in practice there is some 'leakiness' in the system because cytokines can affect bystander B cells too.

With macrophages and dendritic cells (Fig. 18.3, step 5(a)) the only significant differences from the above are that all of them can take up the antigen (because

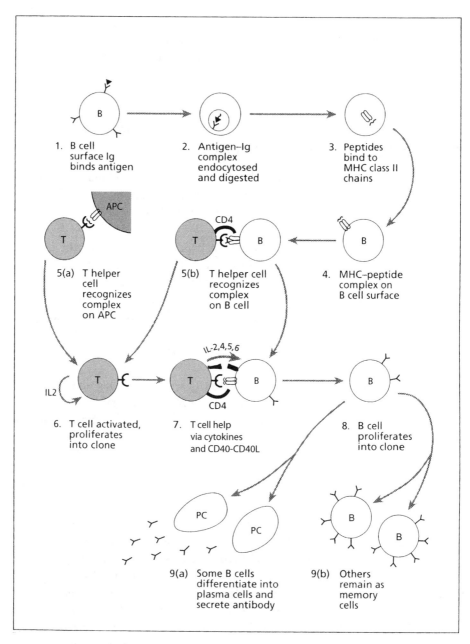

Fig. 18.3 The cellular basis of the antibody response. Both pathways of T cell activation are shown (5a,b). In practice, antigen-presenting dendritic cells (APC) would predominate in the primary response, and B cells in secondary responses.

their recognition is non-specific, see Chapter 10), and that the T cell clone is then available to help either B cells or macrophages. In practice T helper (TH) cells tend to specialize in helping either macrophages (TH1; see Table 17.1 and Fig. 19.6) or B cells (TH2). The effects of T cells on macrophages will be described in Chapter 19; since they do not involve antibody at all, they are referred to as 'cell-mediated'.

Activation of T cells

In Fig. 18.3, steps 5 and 6, T cells are shown becoming activated. As with B cells, T-cell activation requires several signals, of which the most important is recognition of the MHC–peptide complex by the T cell receptor, but interactions between other adhesion and costimulatory molecules are also involved (see Fig. 18.4). When activated, the T cell starts to produce cytokines, particularly IL-2, as well as receptors for IL-2, with the result that the cell stimulates itself to proliferate into a clone and secrete other cytokines needed for, in turn, activating B cells (or macrophages). Note once again the economical way in which, in addition to the actual T–B cell contact-dependent helper mechanisms, non-specific molecules (the cytokines) are made to act only on the right cell by the close proximity that the various receptors and adhesion molecules impose.

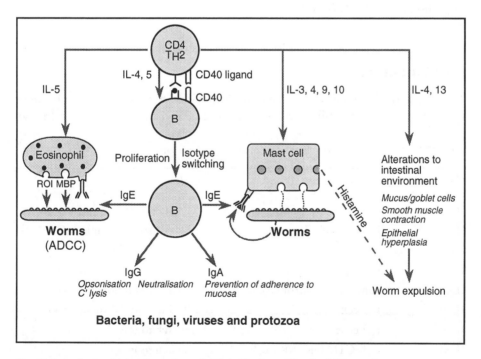

Fig. 18.4 Anti-microbial actions of type 2 CD4+ T cells and B cells. ROI: reactive oxygen intermediates, MBP: major basic protein.

T cell help

In Fig. 18.3, steps 7–9, T cells can be seen helping B cells to proliferate into clones and differentiate into antibody-secreting plasma cells. Help is largely mediated by *cytokines*, IL-2, 4, 5, and 6 being some of the most important secreted T cell products in this case. Some of these cause proliferation, others differentiation, while others again dictate the switch of antibody class (IgM to IgG, IgA, etc.; see Table 18.1), and the generation of memory cells (see below). The latter is a key step, because if all the B cells of a clone were allowed to become plasma cells, which as terminally differentiated cells live only days or weeks, the clone would be lost, and a subsequent response to the same antigen would be seriously impaired. However, because of the remaining memory cells, which are protected from differentiation, subsequent responses are in fact better than primary responses in several respects (Fig. 18.1, Table 18.2). Actual contact between B and T cell is needed for effective help through the interaction of molecules such as CD40 and its ligand on the T cell (CD 154); absence of the latter gives rise to the X-linked hyper IgM syndrome in which B cells fail to switch from IgM to IgG (see Chapter 24).

Thus we see that T cell–B cell interaction is a two-way process: B cells activate T cells to become cells that can help the B cells. Two separate portions of the antigen have to be recognized, with the result that antibody is normally only made against genuinely foreign material. The effect of all these interactions on the fate of pathogens is summarized in Fig. 18.4.

B cell memory

Memory in the immune system compares well with that in the brain; for instance Faroe Islanders were still immune to measles 65 years after the last known

Table 18.1 Cytokines involved in B cell development and function

Cytokine	Source	Effect
IL-2	T cells	Proliferation, IgM secretion
IL-4	T_H2 cells, NKT cells	″ , switch to IgE, IgG
IL-5	T_H2 cells	″ , IgM, IgA
IL-6	T cells, macrophages	Differentiation to plasma cells
IL-7	Bone marrow stromal cells	Early maturation & proliferation
IL-10	T_H2 cells	Proliferation, differentiation
IL-13	T_H2 cells	Switch to IgE
IFNγ	T_H1, CTL, NK, NKT cells	Switch to IgG
TGFβ	T cells	Switch to IgA

Table 18.2 The antibody produced during secondary and subsequent responses differs from primary antibody in several ways, all of which make it more biologically effective

	Primary response	Secondary response
Speed	Slow (days–weeks)	Rapid (1 day)
Duration	Fairly brief (weeks)	Longer (weeks–months)
Amount	Relatively low	High
Ig classes	Mainly IgM at first, with later switch to IgG	Mainly IgG
*Affinity	Variable, medium (but avidity of IgM may be high, owing to multivalency)	High, increases progressively owing to selection of high-affinity B cells and mutation of V genes

* Note the distinction between *affinity* (the strength of binding between a single antigenic determinant and a single antibody combining site) and *avidity* (the strength of the bond between the two whole molecules).

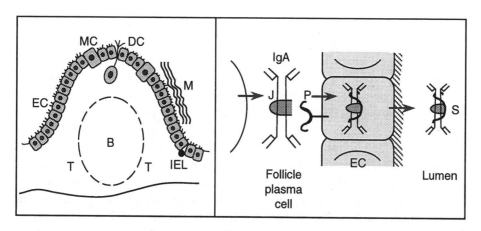

Fig. 18.5 Gut-associated lymphoid tissue, showing (*left*) a subepithelial 'dome' of lymphoid tissue: EC, epithelial cell; MC, microfold cell; DC, dendritic cell; M, layer of mucus; (*right*) how IgA is transported into the gut lumen: P, poly-Ig receptor; S, secretory piece; IEL, intraepithelial lymphocyte.

contact with the virus, and similarly in a US trial antibody to yellow fever virus was still present in the serum nearly 70 years after vaccination. Indeed long-lasting memory is the basis of all successful vaccines. The way in which long-term B cell memory is maintained is discussed in Chapter 20.

The germinal centre

For the most part, all the processes described in this chapter (B cell activation, class switching, affinity maturation, formation of memory cells) occur in special regions of lymphoid tissue known as germinal centres (one is shown diagrammatically in Fig. 15.2). Germinal centres are common in lymph nodes, but can develop wherever there are accumulations of lymphoid tissue. It is the resident *follicular dendritic cells* in germinal centres, specialized for trapping and retaining antigen in the form of complexes with antibody and complement, that regulate B cell activation and the development of memory.

Antibody responses at mucosal surfaces

Though pathogens may enter the tissues through wounds, insect bites, etc. (see Chapter 9), the great majority gain entry across the mucous membranes of the respiratory and gastro-intestinal system. Therefore it is not surprising that the *mucosal immune system* comprises over 50% of all the lymphocytes in the body and two-thirds of all B lymphocytes secrete IgA, the antibody class specialized for protection of mucous surfaces. *Mucosa-associated lymphoid tissue* (MALT) is found in the *gut* (GALT), *bronchi* (BALT), nasopharynx, and genito-urinary system. The most thoroughly studied is the GALT, which also has the most complex task—to mount responses that prevent entry of intestinal pathogens without making responses against the normal gut flora or against food antigens, and without inducing excessive inflammation. How this is managed is still not fully understood; probably pattern-recognition by macrophages and dendritic cells as well as suppressive T cell-derived cytokines such as IL-10 and TGFβ are involved. The essential components of GALT are (1) *lymphoid aggregates* such as the Peyer's patches, where T and B lymphocytes encounter antigens transported across the epithelial layer by microfold cells and dendritic cells, and (2) the *diffuse lymphoid regions* of the villous lamina propria to which these lymphocytes 'home' after entering the circulation (Fig. 18.5). Lamina propria lymphocytes are mainly memory T cells (see Chapter 19) and B cells secreting IgA under the influence of the cytokine TGFβ. Secreted IgA has the advantage of (1) surviving in the proteolytic environment of the gut lumen, and (2) not promoting inflammation, since it does not activate complement or mast cells; its role is to block attachment of pathogens to the epithelium and to export those that penetrate the epithelial barrier.

19 Cell-mediated responses

In this chapter we look at those T cell responses that do not involve B cells and antibody. As Table 17.1 indicated, they are of two distinct kinds, which will need to be considered separately. One type, the activation of macrophages by CD4 (helper) T cells, has many points of resemblance to the activation of B cells, and will be dealt with first. The other, the CD8 (cytotoxic) T cell response, is very different (see later). They do, however, have features in common. Both involve the selection and expansion of *clones* of effector cells from a tiny number of precursors and both result in the long-term survival of a population of *memory* cells that ensure a more vigorous secondary response to the same pathogen—just as B cells do. First we will consider how T cells become activated for these responses. Note that they are referred to as 'cell-mediated' purely for convenience to distinguish them from 'antibody-mediated' B cell responses; in fact, of course, all immune responses originate in *cells*.

T cell activation

There is one important difference between T cell and B cell responses, in that while the B cell product (the antibody molecule) can travel anywhere in the body and has a lifespan of weeks, T cells and their cytokines (see Table 19.1) act transiently and primarily at very short range; thus T cells themselves need to travel to where the pathogen is, or at least close enough to encounter its antigens. These are most likely to be at one of the major sites of pathogen entry—the epithelium of skin and the mucous membranes of the gut, lungs, etc. Here specialized *dendritic cells* take up the pathogen or its antigens and migrate to the local lymph nodes. In the skin it is the Langerhans cells that do this, detaching from the skin during inflammatory responses, migrating via lymphatics to settle in the paracortex of the node where they will eventually encounter, among the ceaselessly passing T cells, those with the appropriate receptor.

The migration of T cells out of the blood vessels to a site of infection is in turn promoted by inflammatory products ('chemokines') and increased expression of adhesion molecules on the vascular endothelium at the site of infection. Local inflammation is also responsible for switching the dendritic cells to an active state

Table 19.1 Cytokines involved in T cell development and function

Cytokine	Source	Effect
IL-2	T cells	T cell proliferation, enhances cytokine production; NK cell activation and growth; B cell proliferation
IL-3	CD4 T cells	Promotes haemopoiesis; mast cell growth and development
IL-4	Th2 CD4 T cells Mast cells	Promotes Th2 differentiation/proliferation; B cell IgE, macrophage inhibition.
IL-5	Th2 CD4 T cells	Eosinophil production & activation, B cell growth, IgM, IgA
IL-7	Bone marrow stroma	Maturation/proliferation of precursor lymphocytes; proliferation of naïve T cells
IL-10	CD4 T cells (Treg and Th2 > Th1), macrophages, DC	Inhibition of macrophage and DC activation (eg. IL-12 secretion and induction of MHC II)
IL-12	Macrophages, DC neutrophils	Promotes Th1 CD4 T cell differentiation and NK cell/T cell IFNγ secretion and cytotoxic activity
IL-13	Th2 CD4 T cells	Mucus production by epithelium, B cell IgE, macrophage inhibition
IL-15	Macrophages etc	NK cell and CD8 T cell proliferation (maintenance of memory T cells)
IL-17	Memory & activated T cells	Induces production of chemokines, TNF & IL-1
IL-18	Macrophages, DC	Promotes Th2 (alone) but Th1 T cells with IL-12; secretion of IFNγ by NK, Th1 & memory CD8 T cells (with IL-12)
IL-23	Macrophages, DC	Inflammation, proliferation of memory CD4 T cells, IFNγ production/Th1 differentiation
IL-27	Macrophage, DC	Proliferation of naïve T cells, IFNγ secretion
IFNγ	Th1 CD4 T cells, CD8 T cells, NK, NK T, γ δ T cells	Macrophage activation; B cell class switching (eg IgG2a); Th1 differentiation; APC activation (eg Class II expression)
TGFβ	T cells, macrophages etc	Inhibits T cell proliferation and function; promotes IgA; inhibits macrophages.
Lymphotoxin	T cells	Neutrophil recruitment/activation; lymphoid organ development

capable of full antigen processing and presentation (see Chapter 18). The precise mixture of pro-inflammatory mediators released by dendritic cells is a major influence on which type of T cell response is initiated—a good example of the subtle interplay between innate and adaptive immunity. The key involvement of local inflammation helps to restrict T cell activity to the site of infection, and in particular to minimize the activation of any T cells that might recognize 'self' peptides.

Note that the above emphasis on dendritic cells applies particularly to primary responses; in subsequent responses involving mainly memory T cells, macrophages and B cells also become important sources of T cell activation (Fig. 19.1).

Effector functions 1: activation of macrophages

Here the macrophage plays a role analogous to that of the B cell in the previous chapter, conveying antigenic peptides from inside the cell to the surface via MHC class II molecules (Fig. 19.2). However, the aim is not to stimulate it to make antibody (which only B cells can do) but to *kill*, or least *control*, the intracellular microbe from which the peptides are derived. As in the case of B cells, 'help' from the CD4 T cell (TH1 variety) consists of various cytokines, the most important here being IFNγ. The need for this help arises because so many microbes are able

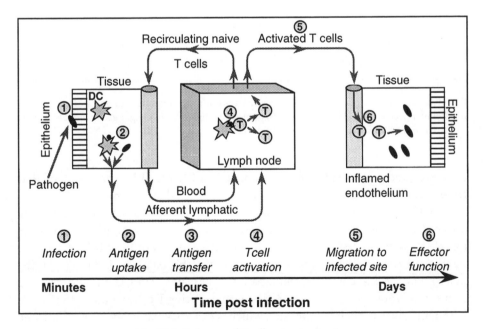

Fig. 19.1 Pathways of T cell activation *in vivo*.

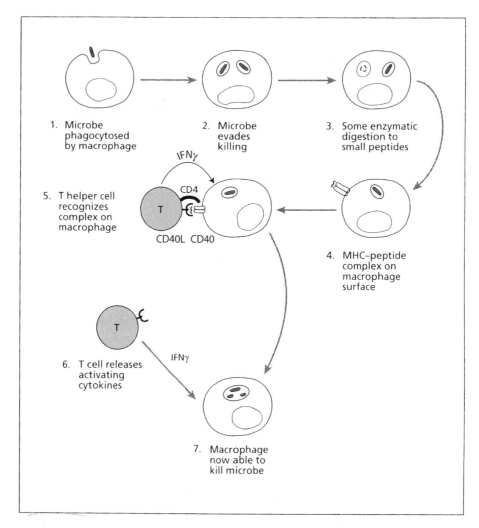

Fig. 19.2 Activation of macrophages by T cells. The same general mechanism operates for intracellular bacteria (e.g. TB), fungi (e.g. *Histoplasma*), and protozoa (e.g. *Leishmania*). Note the similarity to the B cell activation pathway (Fig. 18.4).

to survive and grow inside the macrophage (see Chapter 12 to be reminded that these include some important bacterial and protozoal infections).

A vivid example of how valuable T cell help can be to macrophages is the effect of IFNγ on the protozoon *Leishmania in vitro*. Normal macrophages are unable to stop this pathogen growing, but a few drops of pure IFNγ, followed by the microbial trigger, are sufficient to tip the balance in favour of the macrophage, with complete killing of the parasite. Translated into real-life terms, this would suggest that patients with defective T cells would suffer worse leishmaniasis than their neighbours, which is exactly what is observed. The same goes for TB, leprosy, toxoplasmosis, and many other intracellular infections. The explosion of TB in the tropics in recent years is largely associated with immuno-suppression of CD4 T cells by the AIDS virus HIV. The well-known BCG vaccine, which causes no more than a transient skin lesion in healthy people, can lead to disseminated infection and even death in someone with deficient T cell immunity. While IFNγ remains the major macrophage-activation element, there are also cell-contact-mediated processes just as there are for T–B cell cooperation. In addition, exposure of macrophages to other cytokines or signals (such as IL-4 and IL-13) leads to an 'alternative' activation state with increased expression of the mannose receptor and distinct immunological functions.

The ability of a macrophage, however strongly stimulated, to kill an intracellular microbe or one it has phagocytosed depends on the possession of the appropriate killing machinery. Fortunately, activated macrophages are well armed with both oxidative and non-oxidative mechanisms (see Chapter 11), but many pathogens can resist one or other of these (Chapter 12 and Table 12.1), and even when there is some degree of control of the pathogen, the balance is often quite precarious. A good example is the tendency of long-healed TB lesions to break down and cause a flare-up in people who become run-down—from malnutrition, drugs, diabetes, etc.

Granulomas and chronic inflammation

The mechanisms described so far refer to the activation of individual cells. But in real life there is likely to be extensive recruitment of macrophage precursors (monocytes) as well as PMNs to the site of infection, where they mature and become activated. Unless the pathogen is eliminated quickly these will develop into an organized mass of tissue with macrophages at its centre, some of which may fuse to form giant cells, with surrounding CD4 and CD8 T cells. This is known as a *granuloma*. The T cells, by secreting cytokines, will recruit further cells to the lesion. In the absence of T cells (e.g. in T cell-deprived mice) some macrophage recruitment can occur via NK cell-derived cytokines, but true granulomas do not form. TB, syphilis, and the liver stage of the blood-fluke *Schistosoma* are examples where either killing or 'walling off' of the pathogen is achieved in this way, though granulomas can also be caused by non-microbial but indigestible substances such as asbestos, metals, etc. The mechanism of granuloma formation in tuberculosis is illustrated in Fig. 19.3. Unfortunately, granuloma formation, as well as being beneficial to the host, can also be dangerous. For example, the granulomas surrounding *Schistosoma* eggs can coalesce and block off the circulation of portal blood through the liver, with disastrous results. This is an example of *immunopathology*, which will be dealt with in more detail in Chapter 22.

Activation of other cells by T cells

As well as macrophages, other cells can benefit from T cell-derived cytokines. These include eosinophils, PMNs, natural killer cells, and the haemopoietic cells

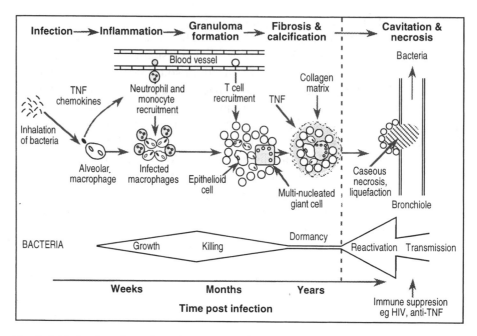

Fig. 19.3 Mechanism of granuloma formation in tuberculosis. Small numbers of bacteria can remain for decades under active control by the immune response; immunosuppression leads to reactivation and transmission of the bacteria. Some infected individuals go directly to acute, necrotic disease.

in the bone marrow. Indeed, so important are T helper cells in regulating the function of other cells that they are sometimes regarded as the 'brains' of the immune system—though this does not do justice to the dendritic cells from which T cells in their turn receive important 'instructions'.

Effector functions 2: cytotoxicity

Viruses differ from most bacteria and higher microorganisms in that they infect and replicate in cells of almost every kind, including many where T cell help would be of no value. For example, a liver cell infected with hepatitis B virus could not kill the virus even if helped, since liver cells lack virus-killing mechanisms. One solution is for a neighbouring cell to make the antiviral cytokine interferon (see Chapter 11). Another somewhat more drastic approach is to kill both the virus and the liver cell. Cytotoxic T cells (CTLs) are specialized for this purpose. They are predominantly CD8 T cells designed to recognize viral peptides bound to MHC class I antigens (see Fig. 19.4) and to destroy all cells carrying that combination. This is made possible by the fact that (1) all nucleated cells carry MHC class I molecules, and (2) the CTL carries CD8 molecules, which recognize MHC class I molecules. Proof that this occurs in any given virus infection is quite hard to obtain, but one clear example is the killing of B lymphocytes infected with Epstein–Barr virus during glandular fever; the CTLs that

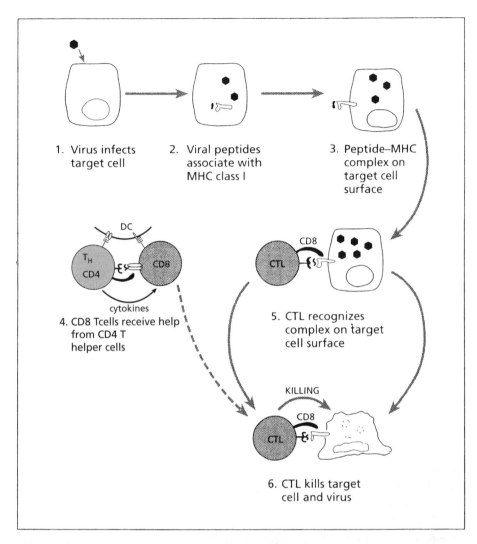

Fig. 19.4 Killing of virus-infected cells by cytotoxic T lymphocytes (CTLs). Note the involvement of different MHC molecules (Class I) and T cell surface molecules (CD8) from those used in the other T cell-mediated responses (compare with Fig 19.2). Generation of effector CTL requires involvement of antigen presenting cells and CD4 T helper cells.

do this were once thought to be 'atypical monocytes', whence the alternative name 'infectious mononucleosis'. Note that T cell-mediated cytotoxicity is the only exception to the rule that T cells work by influencing the 'effector' functions of other cells.

CTLs kill in two related ways: (1) the transfer of granule-derived enzymes ('granzymes') via the actions of perforin into the target cell cytoplasm where they activate the caspase enzymes that in turn induce *apoptosis* or 'cell suicide'; (2) apoptosis can also be triggered via a surface molecule called Fas (the 'death

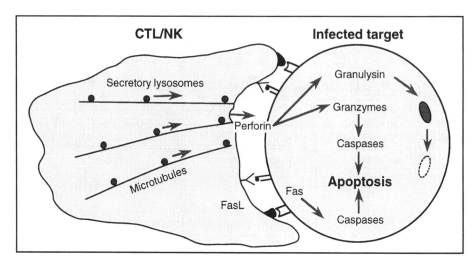

Fig. 19.5 Pathways of cell killing by CTLs and NK cells. Target recognition causes secretory lysosomes to traffic to the contact site along microtubules within the CTL/NK cell. Transfer of granzymes (or cell surface ligation of Fas : FasL) induces target cell apoptosis while the antimicrobial peptide granulysin kills intracellular pathogens such as *M. tuberculosis*.

receptor') with which CTLs can interact via a complementary molecule called Fas ligand. CTLs are 'serial killers'; binding and release of cytotoxic mediators and killing of the target occurs in minutes, allowing the CTL to disengage and search out another victim. Interestingly, the same mechanisms are used by NK cells, though these employ a completely different recognition system (see Fig. 19.5 and Chapter 11). This is fortunate because one of the numerous ways in which viruses attempt to escape CTLs is by inhibiting MHC class I expression, which would render CTLs ineffective but NK cells more effective! Other viral escape strategies include inhibition of caspases, Fas, and other parts of the apoptotic pathway (see Chapter 21).

Although CTLs are chiefly important in virus infections, they probably also act against other intracellular infections such as tuberculosis and malaria (liver stage). In the case of leprosy bacilli that infect the Schwann cells lining peripheral nerves, killing these could be counter-productive if it resulted in the liberation of still living bacilli, which would then have to be dealt with by macrophages. CTLs are also involved in the rejection of transplants and possibly some tumours. Note that in addition to killing, CTLs can also secrete useful cytokines such as IFNγ and it is not always possible to establish which function is the most important in a given infection.

T cell memory

The immunity that follows viral infections such as mumps, measles, rubella, or smallpox, is thought to involve both B and T cells. Experiments suggest that memory T cells can persist for many years, though whether this can occur in the complete absence of antigen is very hard to prove. Certainly the generally longer-lasting protection from live than from killed vaccines, and the reported waning of protection against TB as BCG gradually disappears, suggest a role for antigen persistence. This point is further discussed in Chapters 20 and 27.

T-cell responses at mucosal surfaces

Just as with antibody, T cells may be required to act against pathogens that attempt to enter via the intestinal or respiratory routes. The lamina propria (see Chapter 18) contains CD4, NK, and memory CD8 T cells, which have been shown experimentally to contribute to protection against intestinal viruses, e.g. rotavirus. Moreover, oral vaccines prime this population while systemically injected ones do not, illustrating the specific homing pattern of gut-derived lymphocytes (see Chapter 27) and the importance of delivering vaccines by the right route. Intraepithelial lymphocytes (see Fig. 18.6) also include γδ, and both CD4 and CD8 T cells, the latter possibly being responsible for the induction of tolerance to food antigens.

T$_H$1 and T$_H$2 cells

The distinction between CD4 (helper) T cells that secrete macrophage-activating cytokines such as IFNγ and those that activate B cells with cytokines such as IL-

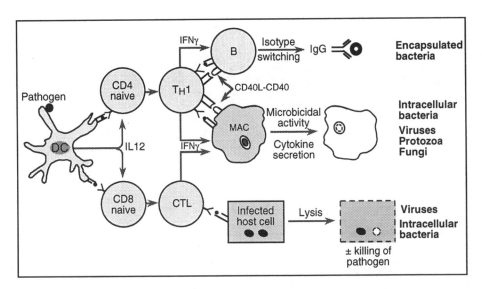

Fig. 19.6 Anti-microbial activities of Type 1 T cell responses.

4, 5, 10, 13 has been mentioned several times (see Table 18.1). In general, the T_H subset activated is appropriate to the type of infection—T_H1 for intracellular pathogens where macrophage activation is required (Fig. 19.6) and T_H2 for antibody responses to deal with extracellular pathogens, with further specialization towards particular subclasses, e.g. IgA for intestinal infections and IgE for helminths. T_H1 and T_H2 cells develop from a common precursor (T_H0) and the stimulus to their differentiation comes mainly from cytokines of the innate immune system. IL-12 (from dendritic cells, macrophages, and PMNs) favours the T_H1, and IL-4 the T_H2 pathway. Since both populations secrete cytokines that tend to self-perpetuate their own population and suppress the other, responses usually remain predominantly of one or the other type, even when this is not the most appropriate (see Chapter 21 for examples of this from leprosy and EBV infection).

20 Regulation of immune responses and memory

Like most physiological processes, immune responses have the potential to damage their host unless properly regulated. In the case of innate immunity (complement, phagocytes, etc.; see Chapter 11) this is mainly a question of avoiding excessive responses and of focusing them as accurately as possible on the right (that is, the *foreign*) target. Often, however, some 'overspill' is unavoidable, as is shown, for example, by the inflammation and tissue damage that frequently accompany the elimination of a pathogen.

With adaptive responses there is the whole new problem of *lymphocyte proliferation*. The Persian legend of the grains of rice on the chessboard—one grain on the first square, two on the second, four on the next, and so on, culminating in a pile of rice weighing about 100 000 000 000 tons—gives a chilling idea of what could happen if clonal expansion of a B or T lymphocyte carried on unchecked. Several obvious factors would prevent this calamity, lack of available space and nutrients, for example. But Nature has seen to it that more subtle processes act to regulate the size of lymphocyte responses to somewhere near the optimum, that is, large enough to eliminate the pathogen if that is possible, but small enough to allow responses to other pathogens at the same time, with the added bonus of retaining *memory* to each one and mounting a stronger response if it reappears. In this chapter we review these regulatory processes, and we also consider some aspects of memory that have not already been discussed in Chapters 18 and 19.

We can distinguish four levels of control:

(1) *Elimination* of antigen: since antigen is a requirement for the initiation of lymphocyte proliferation, the latter will tend to diminish as antigen disappears.

(2) Once a population of lymphocytes has responded, the majority of them (more than 90%) will die by *apoptosis*. Those that survive will become memory cells.

(3) Lymphocytes carry surface *receptors* which when ligated can induce inhibition of proliferation and/or function, particularly of B cells.

(4) Lymphocytes can inhibit each other—the concept of *regulatory* (mainly T) *cells*.

Elimination of antigen

Since the end-result of a successful response, whether by B cells, T cells, or both, is the elimination of the inducing pathogen and therefore of its antigens, and since antigen is an essential part of the triggering process, a completely successful response does not really need to be turned off; it will simply die away as antigen disappears. Thus the rise and fall of an antibody response can be seen partly as an expression of antigen availability. However, as will be described in the following chapter, many successful pathogens have evolved strategies for avoiding complete elimination, while others recur so frequently that their antigens are present for months or years at a time. In such cases alternative means are required to avoid the 'chessboard' scenario.

Apoptosis

The elimination of antigen-specific lymphocytes occurs by *apoptosis* (also known as 'programmed cell death' or 'cell suicide'). Unlike *necrosis*, this induces very little inflammation and is a normal part of all immune responses. Previously activated effector cells are particularly susceptible. The process is induced by a variety of stimuli, including TNF, TGFβ, APO-1/Fas, and reduction of the 'survival' protein Bcl-2. Apoptotic cells shrink in size, with a characteristic 'laddering' of DNA, and break into small fragments that are removed by phagocytes.

Inhibitory receptors

The most striking example of receptor-mediated inhibition is the interaction between antigen–antibody complexes and the receptor on B cells known as FcγR II or CD32. When the IgG of an antigen–antibody complex binds to this molecule and at the same time the antigen binds to the B-cell Ig, an inhibitory signal is generated. This mechanism is referred to as *antibody feedback*. Clearly such a mechanism will not come into play until substantial amounts of IgG have been made and have bound to the antigen. Antibody feedback has important consequences, including: (1) the tendency of maternally derived IgG to inhibit antibody responses by the newborn—which is why vaccination is usually delayed (see Chapter 27), and (2) the prevention of Rhesus sensitization in RhD− mothers by RhD+ infants; anti-RhD antibody being given immediately after birth to inhibit further anti-RhD antibody formation.

Other examples of receptor-mediated inhibition include the KIR receptors found on NK and T cells (see Chapter 11 and Fig. 11.9), and the molecules induced on T cells after activation, such as CTLA-4, which binds to B7 on antigen-presenting cells and gives the T cell an inhibitory signal to dampen down the response. The cytotoxic apparatus of CD8 T cells (see Chapter 19) may also have a regulatory role, since defects of perforins and lysosomal movement lead to overactive antiviral T cell responses.

Regulation by T cells

This term covers two distinct kinds of cell: (1) T cells that are stimulatory for one type of immune response but inhibitory for another, and (2) T cells which are purely inhibitory. Both kinds operate through selective release of cytokines.

Type 1 and type 2 T cells

Type 1 and 2 helper cells have already been mentioned in Chapters 17 and 19, and Fig. 20.1 emphasizes their principal difference, namely that T$_H$1 cells secrete cytokines such as IFNγ, whose main stimulatory effects are on macrophages, while T$_H$2 cells secrete cytokines such as IL-4, which stimulate B cells. Thus T$_H$1 cells are active in cell-mediated responses and T$_H$2 in antibody responses. In addition, type 1 cytokines inhibit the generation and activity of type 2 cells and vice versa, which probably helps to ensure that responses are polarized towards antibody or cell-mediated immunity. Not only CD4 but also CD8 T cells show this pattern of cytokines.

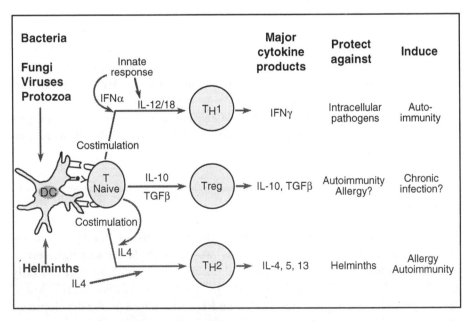

Fig. 20.1 Lineage decisions of CD4 T cells. Naïve CD4 T cells can differentiate into either TH1, TH2 or regulatory T cells (Treg) according to the conditions present during antigen presentation.

Regulatory T cells

This population, whose separate existence as *suppressor T cells* was debated for many years was more recently confirmed in relation to the prevention of autoimmunity (see Chapter 23) and now referred to as *regulatory T cells*. They appear to have mostly inhibitory functions, via either cell contact or cytokines such as IL-10 and TGFβ (Fig. 20.1). Induction of these cells can be a survival strategy for some pathogens such as *Leishmania*.

Therapeutic regulation

There are occasions when it may be necessary to deliberately down-regulate an immune response, most commonly by the use of *immunosuppressive* drugs. Reasons for immunosuppression include the hypersensitivity conditions to be described in Chapter 22 (allergies, granulomas, etc.), autoimmunity (Chapter 23). and, of course, the special situation of organ transplantation. As far as infectious disease is concerned, the major indication for inhibiting immunity is the excessive cell-mediated immune responses found in chronic diseases such as tuberculosis, which in their efforts to kill and/or wall off the pathogen may end up destroying whole organs. In the case of allergies, it is usually more effective to inhibit the innate mechanisms actually causing the damage—mast cells, histamine, etc. When pathology can be shown to be due to excessive cytokine activity, it might be possible to block or neutralize this; an example is the use of drugs or antibodies against TNF in conditions associated with bacterial endotoxins—with little success so far. But in general, immunosuppression is likely to lay the patient open to *more* rather than *less* danger from infection. Table 20.1 lists the most commonly used therapies.

On the other hand, an inadequate immune response may benefit from being *enhanced*. Cytokines have been tried (e.g. IFN and IL-2 for chronic intracellular infections and some tumours), but there is suggestive evidence that various regimes (diet supplements, physical and even mental disciplines, etc.) may be beneficial too, though hard evidence is usually lacking. For enhancing antigen-specific responses, *vaccination* has proved so effective that it is given its own chapter (Chapter 27).

Memory

The generation of specific memory is one of the major virtues of adaptive immunity, ensuring that an individual responds progressively faster and more effectively with repeated exposure to a particular pathogen. It explains why one only gets diseases like measles once, and also why the measles vaccine works. Memory is a property of lymphocytes, both B and T, and is based on the development of *memory cells*, which differ in a number of ways from the B and T cells they are derived from (Table 20.2).

Table 20.1 Some commonly used immunosuppressive therapies

Drug/method	Target of action	Main applications
Corticosteroids	Cytokines (IL-1,6; TNF); Cell migration Inflammation	Hypersensitivities Autoimmunity
Cyclophosphamide	B cells	Autoimmunity
Azathioprine	Cell division	Organ grafting
Cyclosporin; FK 506	IL-2 (i.e. T cell activation)	″ ″
Anti-lymphocyte antibodies (e.g. CD3)	Lymphocytes	″ ″
Anti-cytokine antibodies (e.g. TNFα)	Cytokines	Rheumatoid arthritis, Crohn's disease
Antihistamines	Histamine	Allergies
Sodium cromoglycate	Mast cells	″

Table 20.2 Naïve, effector, and memory lymphocytes compared

	Naïve	Effector	Memory
B cells			
Location	Secondary lymphoid organs	Germinal centre Bone marrow	Secondary lymphoid organs
Surface markers	IgM, IgD	Low Ig; MHC II	IgG, IgA, IgE
Activity	Minimal	Ig secretion Proliferation	Minimal—but rapid response on re-exposure
T cells			
Location	Secondary lymphoid organs (recirculating)	Sites of infection	Recirculating gut, lung
Surface markers	CD44 low, CD45RA CD62L high CCR7 high	CD44 high, CD45RO CD62L low CCR7 low	CD44 high, CD45RO CD62L high or low CCR7 high or low
Activity	Minimal	Proliferation Cytotoxicity Cytokine secretion	Minimal—but rapid response on re-exposure

Generation of memory cells

We have already stressed what the results would be if all the possible progeny of a proliferating lymphocyte clone survived (the 'chessboard' scenario) and described how in fact most of them eventually die. However, the opposite extreme would be equally disastrous, because if *all* of them died, the individual would then be left with no lymphocytes of the relevant specificity and would thus be specifically unresponsive, or *tolerant*, to that particular pathogen, and worse off than before. Mechanisms therefore exist to prevent this, as follows.

B cells

As already mentioned in earlier chapters, neither Ig molecules nor individual plasma cells normally survive more than a matter of weeks. However, plasma cells in the *bone marrow* can produce antibody for many months whilst memory cells in secondary lymphoid organs, though not making antibody, are maintained for decades. Thus some antibody is immediately available to deal with a second infection, and more can be made within a few days. It is still controversial whether or not the survival of memory cells requires the continued presence of small amounts of antigen, for example in the form of immune complexes on follicular dendritic cells. Experiments in mice suggest that memory cells can indeed survive in the complete absence of antigen. (But mice do not last for 75 years as human memory does! See Chapter 18.) In favour of the idea of antigen persistence is that many pathogens are known to survive virtually indefinitely even in immune hosts, and that living viral vaccines often induce longer-lasting memory than killed ones, but another possible mechanism would be 'boosting' by cross-reaction between the antigens in question and other molecules in the environment.

T cells

Memory T cells appear to be a heterogeneous population with slightly different histories. (1) Due to the limited availability of essential stimuli such as antigen-presenting cells and cytokines, some T cells proliferate but do not go through full differentiation and remain as long-lived memory cells, recirculating through lymphoid organs just like naïve cells and inactive until re-exposed to the same pathogen. (2) A second population consists of cells that have functioned but survive for some time at the original site of infection (e.g. lung, gut) ready to respond to a subsequent infection, though only in the relatively short term. Because of differences in surface molecules (adhesion molecules, chemokine receptors) both types of cell can respond more rapidly than naïve T cells. However, T cell responses do not appear to be prolonged in the manner described above for B cells.

Whatever the exact mechanism, the question of how multiple pools of memory cells to dozens or hundreds of different antigens are maintained at a reasonably constant size is a fascinating one. Presumably as new memory cells are generated others die, perhaps through competition for critical growth factors or other survival signals, but one can only marvel at the precision of the homeostatic mechanisms involved.

Activation and response by memory cells

B cells

The superiority of secondary antibody responses is due to four properties of memory as compared to naïve B cells: (1) there are more of them specific for the antigen in question; (2) they differentiate into plasma cells more rapidly; (3) during the primary response, most of them switch from making the IgM isotype to IgG (or IgA); once switched, they remain as IgG or IgA producers from the start of the secondary response; (4) because of the high frequency of somatic mutation in the Ig genes during B cell proliferation (mainly in germinal centres), a few cells emerge whose antibody has higher affinity for the inducing antigen. As antigen levels decline, these cells are preferentially selected for stimulation, so that the average affinity of the total antibody population rises ('matures'), sometimes by up to 100-fold. Both isotype switching and proliferation are greatly helped by T cells, so that high-affinity IgG tends to be made predominantly against protein antigens.

T cells

Memory T cells can be activated in three different ways. (1) By the same pathogen as that encountered before; note, however, that T cells do not show class switching or somatic mutation. (2) By a different pathogen which shares one or more antigens with the original inducing one, resulting in a secondary-type response to what should theoretically be a primary infection. This is known as *cross-reactive* or *heterologous* immunity, and could have important consequences as one ages and accumulates T memory populations, enhancing one's response to a new pathogen in a way that might be beneficial (more rapid elimination) or harmful (more immunopathology, see Chapter 22). An example may be the curious fact that responses to one strain of influenza virus often consist mainly of activity against the strain first encountered, perhaps many years ago ('original antigenic sin'). (3) Unlike naïve T cells, memory cells can be activated by high local levels of cytokines induced by completely unrelated pathogens; this is called *bystander* activation and is particularly a feature of memory CD8 T cells, which can be driven by IL-12 and IL-18 to secrete large amounts of IFNγ. This differs from (1) and (2) above, in being independent of the T cell receptor (TCR).

Maintenance of memory cells

Here the key question is whether long-lived *antigen* is needed to maintain long-lived *memory*. Only by being able to detect every single molecule of an antigen in the body—an impossible task—could this question be settled definitely, but cell-transfer experiments in mice suggest that while antigen certainly helps to keep memory up to optimal levels, it may not be strictly required; possibly cytokines such as IL-15 may be sufficient, as in (3) above.

21 How pathogens escape adaptive immunity

As the last five chapters have stressed, the keynote of adaptive immunity is the very high *specificity of recognition*. As compared to the relatively few pattern-recognizing receptors of innate immunity, B and T lymphocyte receptors can be generated to recognize a virtually infinite range of foreign molecules; it is certainly impossible to imagine a pathogen *none* of whose antigens would be recognized. Would-be successful parasites must therefore evolve ways of avoiding this recognition, in addition to those ways, already discussed in Chapter 12, of avoiding the disposal mechanisms of the innate immune system.

Every pathogen has its own approach to the problem of being recognized by B and T cells, but they can be grouped into three main categories:

(1) attempts to *conceal* their presence from lymphocytes;

(2) *variation* of surface antigens;

(3) *suppression* or *modulation* of lymphocytes or lymphocyte function.

Concealment

Anything that intervenes between a microbial antigen and a B or T cell capable of recognizing it will obviously reduce the chances of inducing an immune response, or of restimulating already existing memory cells. Three fairly common things that can do this are:

(1) cell membranes (the pathogen resides inside host cells);

(2) cysts, usually of host origin, induced by the pathogen;

(3) host-derived molecules taken up by the pathogen (and mimicry of host antigens by the pathogen).

Intracellular residence

Microbes that survive inside host cells are effectively protected against recognition by B lymphocytes, but as explained in Chapters 17 and 19, the MHC system betrays their presence to T lymphocytes and especially to the CD8 killers (Fig. 21.1). Viruses, in particular, have evolved a number of ways round this. They

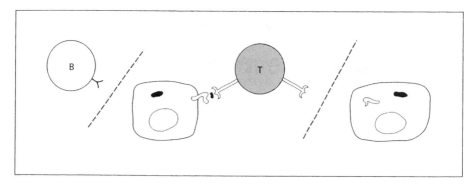

Fig. 21.1 An intracellular habitat protects against recognition by B cells. To avoid recognition by T cells, an intracellular pathogen must inhibit the function of MHC molecules.

may interfere with the generation of MHC molecules in the endoplasmic reticulum, their transport to the cell surface, or their maintenance there (e.g. CMV, EBV, adenovirus, herpesvirus); alternatively they may prevent the host cell being killed by CTLs by inhibiting the caspase enzymes and other mechanisms leading to apoptosis (e.g. myxoma). Not only viruses but also larger pathogens such as *Chlamydia, Yersinia, Coxiella, Leishmania,* and TB can inhibit MHC and CD1 expression, costimulation, cytokine release, apoptosis, and indeed virtually anything that could lead to their demise. It is remarkable that in almost every case, successful pathogens rely on more than one single escape mechanism (see Table 12.1).

One vulnerable point in the life of an intracellular pathogen occurs when it attempts to spread to other cells or to infect another individual and is exposed to immune elements in blood or tissue fluid. The bacterium *Listeria monocytogenes* avoids this by the simple strategy of: (1) lysing the membrane of the phagosome in which it resides to enter the cytoplasm, and (2) causing a protrusion of the cell membrane to push into a neighbouring cell, which then buds off to leave the organism in a new phagosome, having never been exposed to the outside of any cell. Some viruses can pass directly into the outside world by shedding into structures that 'face outwards', for example the gut or the skin and its glands. Others do not spread at all but are content to reside, after a brief infection, in long-lived cells, e.g. varicella-zoster (chickenpox) in the central nervous system, from which it can emerge decades later to cause a new skin infection (shingles). One could perhaps regard the DNA of the host cell as the safest hiding place of all; this is where retroviruses such as HIV persist so disastrously. Worse, one of the major sites of HIV growth is in the T cells and macrophages of the immune system itself (see *immunosuppression,* below).

Cysts

Cysts are a feature of some worm infections. Initially the cyst is of worm origin, but induces inflammation in surrounding tissue, with fibrosis and even calcifica-

Table 21.1 Mechanisms of pathogen interference with antigen-presenting cell function

Effect on APC	Examples of organism
Reduced endocytosis	CMV
Inhibition of phago-lysosome fusion or phagosome maturation	*M. tuberculosis*, *Chlamydia*, *Legionella*, *Salmonella*
Reduced MHC Class II synthesis	*M. tuberculosis*, *Chlamydia*, *Toxoplasma*
Impaired MHC trafficking/expression	Cholera toxin, *E. coli* heat labile toxin
Reduced antigen processing	*Salmonella*
Reduced MHC Class I synthesis/expression	*Salmonella*, *Yersinia*, HIV
Inhibition of proteasomes	*Yersinia*, EBV, CMV
Inhibition of TAP	HSV-1,2
Expression of non-functional MHC I-like decoys	CMV
Apoptosis of APC	*Yersinia*
Inhibition of DC maturation	CMV
Over-expression of inhibitory molecules (e.g. IL-10, TGFβ, nitric oxide)	*M. tuberculosis*, *B. pertussis*, *Yersinia*
Impaired IL-12 production	Measles, *Leishmania*, *M. tuberculosis*, HIV
Destruction of lymphoid architecture	*Leishmania*
Reduced expression of CD-1	*M. tuberculosis*
Impaired costimulatory molecule expression	*Leishmania donovani*

tion, so that the main bulk of it is host derived. A striking example is the 'hydatid' cyst of the tapeworm *Echinococcus*, which can grow to enormous size—several quarts of fluid containing millions of immature worms. Escaping worm antigens induce vigorous antibody responses, especially of the IgE class, but these antibodies cannot reach the worms inside the cysts. Instead, if released—e.g. during surgical operation—they bind to mast cells and can precipitate severe allergic reactions (see Chapter 22). The tapeworm *Taenia* and the lung-fluke *Paragonimus* are two other worms that give rise to cysts.

Uptake of host antigens

This is another worm strategy, best illustrated by the blood-fluke *Schistosoma*. The surface of these worms, which live free in the venous circulation and therefore exposed to the entire range of immune components, becomes coated with host-derived molecules, including blood group glycolipids, MHC molecules, immunoglobulins of all kinds, etc. The result is that, as far as the host recognition molecules are concerned, the worm is completely camouflaged and appears as 'self'. This strategy probably works better with slow-growing worms than it would with a rapidly dividing bacterium or protozoon whose surface area doubles every few hours.

Rather different in purpose are the viral genes increasingly being identified that appear to have been acquired from their hosts; these include a remarkable selection of cytokine-like and cytokine receptor-like molecules, presumably of use to the virus in manipulating the immune system for its own purposes (see also *immunosuppression*, below and Table 21.2).

Antigen mimicry

There are several well-established cases where closely similar molecules are found on host cells and on a pathogen, which might be considered an attempt at disguise. A famous example is the myocardium-like antigen on the wall of Group A β-haemolytic streptococci, though this is probably more important as a cause of *autoimmunity* than as an escape mechanism for the pathogen and is dealt with in Chapter 23.

Table 21.2 Some examples of virus-coded cytokine and cytokine receptor homologues

Virus	Cytokine/receptor	Function
Vaccinia	Epidermal growth factor	Cell growth
EBV	IL-10	Anti-inflammatory
CMV	"	Immunosuppressive
HHV8	IL-6	B cell growth
	Viral chemokine	Chemotactic antagonist
HHV6	"	Angiogenic
*HIV	"	Entry into cells
*RSV	"	"
CMV	TNF receptor	Inhibits secreted TNF
Vaccinia	IL-1β receptor	Blocks fever
	IFN α,β,γ receptors	Blocks IFN
HHV8	Viral chemokine receptor	?
CMV	"	?
HHV6	"	?

* RNA viruses; with these exceptions, viral homologues are characteristic of large DNA viruses.

Antigenic variation

This is one of the most cunning of all pathogen strategies, highly effective at confusing the recognition systems of adaptive immunity, and is found in all classes of pathogen from viruses to protozoa. The principle is that by continuously changing the shape of important surface antigens, or the sequence of critical peptides, the pathogen ensures that it induces a series of primary immune responses, rather than increasingly effective secondary responses, by B and T cells.

The classic example is the influenza virus. This RNA virus is covered with protein antigens of two kinds, haemagglutinin and neuraminidase, each of which exists in many different forms, known to virologists by number. Thus an attack of H1N1 ('Spanish') influenza would not protect you against the H2N2 ('Asian') or H3N2 ('Hong Kong') viruses (these are the major human strains). A given strain of virus can change these antigens by mutation, producing minor alterations known as '*antigenic drift*'. Every few years, however, a more drastic change can occur by exchange of RNA between quite different influenza viruses, usually of human and bird origin, the recombination occurring in pigs, which are susceptible to both human and bird strains. This happens mainly in the Far East and is called '*antigenic shift*'. By spreading round the world, these new recombinant viruses ('escape mutants') are responsible for the major pandemics of influenza (Fig. 21.2).

A third type of variation is one that occurs during infection within a single individual, probably driven by the need to escape the immune response. This is a particular feature of the AIDS virus, HIV. Not only does antigenic variation make the development of secondary responses impossible, but it also interferes with the design of vaccines. An ideal flu or HIV vaccine would have to contain all possible variants—a daunting task!

Also occurring during the individual infection is the slightly different type of antigenic variation displayed by the blood-dwelling protozoa that cause sleeping sickness, *Trypanosoma gambiense* and *rhodesiense*. Like schistosome worms, these are at the mercy of all the immune components found in blood. However the DNA of these parasites contains about 1000 quite different genes, each of which codes for a glycoprotein molecule with which the surface of the parasite can be completely coated. By a process of gene copying and translocation, any of these 1000 glycoproteins can be used as a coat protein. When the rapidly dividing trypanosome comes under attack from antibody, its progeny simply switch genes. Thus the host is obliged to make a series of primary responses (Fig. 21.3). Without drug-treatment the disease is fatal, and with so many variants the prospects for a vaccine look fairly slim at present.

Antigenic variation is also a feature of malaria and of several bacterial diseases (e.g. relapsing fever due to *Borrelia recurrentis* and undulant fever due to *Brucella*). The antigenic diversity (or polymorphism) seen in so many pathogens, from adenoviruses and salmonellae to malaria, is simply the end result of

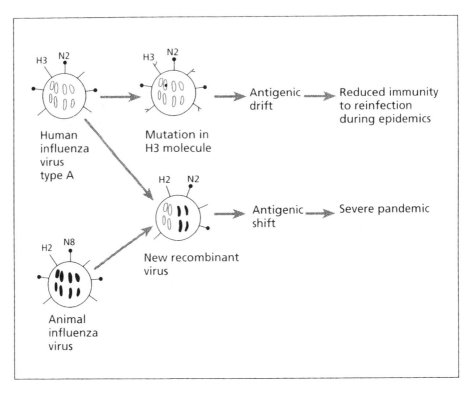

Fig. 21.2 The human influenza A virus is subject to antigenic variation of two kinds: drift (*top*) and shift (*bottom*).

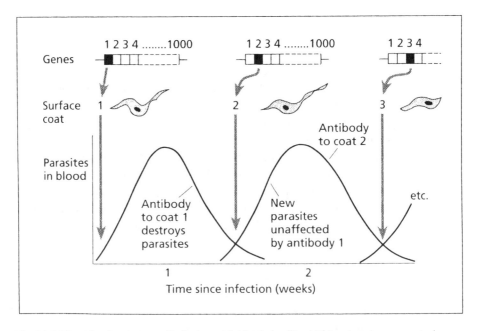

Fig. 21.3 The relapsing pattern of infection with blood-dwelling (African) trypanosomes is due to the repeated appearance and destruction of waves of parasites with completely different surface coat glycoproteins, each requiring a different specificity of antibody for its elimination. The host is thus prevented from developing memory, switching to IgG, etc.

antigenic variation over a time-scale of years, leading to the coexistence of many different variants. For completeness, we should also mention that some pathogens display different antigens at different stages of their life cycle, so that the host may be immune to one stage and not another; a striking example is seen in schistosomiasis, where immunity to new infections by the larval stage allows the adult worms to lead a peaceful and uncrowded existence.

Immunosuppression

During many infectious diseases, patients are found to be immunodeficient to some degree. There may be a reduction of T cells in the blood, or a failure to produce a good antibody response or switch from IgM to IgG (see Chapters 24 and 25). Immunosuppression is seen in measles, mumps, chickenpox, glandular fever, tuberculosis, leprosy, and many protozoal diseases. During measles, skin tests for tuberculosis become negative and susceptibility to a flare-up increases. Quite mild malaria has been shown to severely impair the ability of otherwise normal people to respond to some bacterial vaccines—a very important consideration in terms of public health programmes. Whether it actually helps the malaria parasite to survive is debatable, but there are examples in experimental animals where deletion of an immunosuppressive molecule undoubtedly helps the host to eliminate other infections. The wildly excessive T cell responses induced by staphylococcal and streptococcal superantigens (see Chapter 17) could also be considered as an interference with normal immunity.

The above examples of immunosuppression are normally temporary and probably do no long-term harm. However, some pathogens cause severe and progressive immunosuppression—the classic example being HIV. Here the steady loss of CD4 (helper) T cells leads to a total inability to cope with intracellular parasites including viruses, mycobacteria, fungi, and protozoa. This terrible disease, the commonest infectious cause of immunodeficiency, is discussed in more detail in Chapter 25.

The actual mechanisms involved in immunosuppression are extremely varied. The mimicry of cytokines and cytokine receptors by viruses, already mentioned, probably constitutes a very effective way of avoiding immune attack. It is particularly a feature of herpesviruses, and a striking example is the IL-10-like molecule produced by the Epstein–Barr virus. IL-10 is an extremely suppressive cytokine for cell-mediated immunity. Table 21.2 lists some other representative examples.

Suppression may operate at the level of tissues rather than cells, for instance the loss of germinal centre integrity in the protozoal disease leishmaniasis. Another rather special case is the blockage of normal lymph recirculation by filarial worms in elephantiasis.

Diversion of immune responses

Rather than simply suppressing immunity, some pathogens are able to *divert* the immune response from a type that would harm them to another, harmless type for example by the production of soluble 'decoy' antigens which attract the attention of the immune system away from the pathogen itself (see Table 21.2). Sometimes pathogens survive because the host mounts an ineffective response. Here the classic example is leprosy. This is caused by a mycobacterium similar to the tubercle bacillus, which is susceptible to T-cell-mediated but not antibody-mediated immunity. Many patients appear to achieve protective immunity without serious disease, but for reasons not fully understood, the infection sometimes induces excessive cell-mediated immunity, resulting in destruction of the bacilli and damage to host tissues, and sometimes strong but ineffective antibody responses. These two patterns of response, referred to as *tuberculoid* and *lepromatous*, respectively, represent the extremes of a 'spectrum' (Fig. 21.4), and a

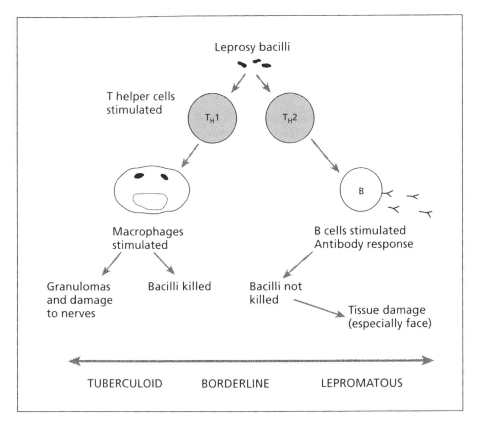

Fig. 21.4 The 'spectrum' seen among leprosy patients may be related to the activities of T helper cell subsets. By releasing different cytokines, T_H1 and T_H2 cells induce completely different patterns of immune response, with different clinical consequences. What determines the choice of T_H1 or T_H2 pathway in different individuals is still unknown.

somewhat similar pattern is seen in cutaneous leishmaniasis. It is suspected that the decisive event is the switching of the helper T cells towards the T_H1 or T_H2 type (see Table 17.1).

Polyclonal activation

Yet another variation on the theme of immunosuppression is the ability of some pathogens to activate large numbers of lymphocytes, most of which will not have the appropriate specificity to attack them. The staphylococcal superantigens that do this to T cells have already been mentioned, and also those T-independent antigens that activate B cells polyclonally such as LPS from Gram-bacteria (see Chapter 18). Many infections, particularly by protozoa such as those causing malaria and trypanosomes, are accompanied by high levels of antibody, much of which is not detectably specific for the pathogen. It is reasonable to suspect (though hard to prove) that these useless lymphocyte responses restrict the host's ability to mount useful responses. Moreover, there is evidence that, because they may include anti-self responses, they may actually induce damage to host tissues. In fact polyclonal lymphocyte activation is believed to be the cause of some *autoimmune diseases* (see Chapter 23).

22 Disease due to adaptive immunity I: hypersensitivity

The way in which lymphocytes respond, amplifying a tiny minority of specific cells into large clones with powerful potential to damage their target, makes it all the more important for the responses to take place against the right target and in the right place. Unfortunately this does not always happen precisely, with the result that host tissues can also be damaged, the actual damage being frequently inflicted by elements of the innate immune system (refer back to Chapter 13 for a reminder of how innate immunity itself can also over-react). Tissue damage caused in this way is called *immunopathology*, or sometimes *hypersensitivity*. If lymphocytes actually start to respond to the host's own (i.e. self) antigens, this is called *autoimmunity*. Autoimmunity is an abnormal response and will be discussed in the following chapter; here we consider the unwelcome side-effects of 'normal' responses against perfectly ordinary non-self antigens.

All over the world, one system of nomenclature is used to classify these effects—the one introduced in 1958 by Gell and Coombs, who divided up the causes of hypersensitivity as shown in Table 22.1.

Type I (allergic) hypersensitivity

This is far the commonest type of immunopathology, since about one person in six suffers from some kind of allergy. The fundamental problem is that IgE antibody can do harm as well as good, triggering off acute inflammatory reactions where they are not needed. Hay fever is an example. Most people can inhale the pollen grains, dust particles, etc. that the air is full of without ill effect, either coughing them up or phagocytosing them. However, some people have the tendency to make large amounts of IgE against a particular animal or plant antigen; their mast cells and basophils pick this up via their Fcε receptors, and when the antigen comes along again, activating the mast cell by cross-linking two or more receptors, the cells degranulate, release a number of preformed mediators (Fig. 22.1 and Table 22.2), and initiate a local inflammatory reaction. Such reactions are called *allergic* and people with this tendency are called *atopic*. As hinted in Chapter 11, inflammation can be most useful in getting blood and blood components to the site of an infection, but if it occurs in the nose and eyes every time

Table 22.1 Mechanisms of hypersensitivity: the Gell and Coombs classification

Type; name	Mediated by	Example
I; *allergic*	IgE antibody and mast cells	Hay fever
II; *cytotoxic*	IgG antibody; complement; phagocytes	Blood transfusion rejection
III; *complex-mediated*	Soluble antigen–antibody complexes; polymorphs; complement	Glomerulonephritis
IV; *cell-mediated*	T cells; cytokines	TB granuloma
V; *stimulatory* (added later)	Antibody to hormone receptors	Thyrotoxicosis

Table 22.2 Mast cell-derived mediators of hypersensitivity

Mediator	Biological effects
Preformed in granules	
Histamine	Vascular permeability increase; bronchoconstriction
Chemotactic factors	Attract PMNs and other cells
Platelet-activating factor	Release of factors causing vascular permeability
Heparin	Anticoagulant
Newly formed after activation	
Prostaglandins	Pain, fever
Leukotrienes	Attract cells

a pollen grain settles there it is just a nuisance. Likewise in the skin (urticaria). If it occurs in the bronchi it can be dangerous, causing attacks of asthma. And if it occurs all over the body it can even be fatal, as very occasionally happens with the *anaphylaxis* following a bee-sting or a penicillin injection.

Despite intensive study, the reasons why one person makes a large amount of IgE to one molecule and a second to another, while a third is not allergic to anything, are not understood, but it has been thought, like the leprosy spectrum (see Fig. 21.4), to be related to the pattern of cytokine production by T helper cells, T_H2 cells favouring allergy by releasing IL-4 and IL-13 and T_H1 cells tending to inhibit this. It is worth mentioning that for IgE 'a large amount' is a relative term, since even a 1000-fold increase in serum level leaves IgE as the minority immunoglobulin class (look back to Table 16.1). To test for allergy, a small amount of the suspected allergen is injected into the skin, and if there is IgE on the local mast cells, a red, swollen 'immediate hypersensitivity' reaction comes up within 10 minutes. Allergy is on the increase in the Western world, but not the tropics, and this has been the subject of much debate (see below).

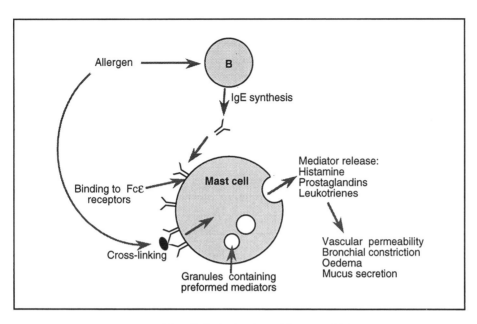

Fig. 22.1 The cellular basis of type 1 hypersensitivity.

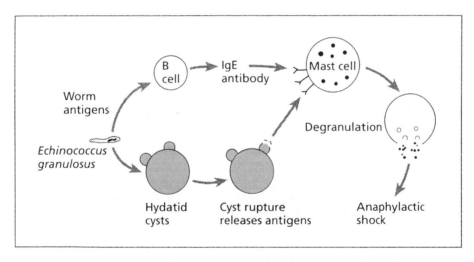

Fig. 22.2 Anaphylaxis, with vascular collapse, following rupture of a hydatid cyst, illustrates the mechanism of type I hypersensitivity. Less severe symptoms, often localized to one organ (e.g. the lung), may occur in other worm infections.

Although most antigens causing allergy (allergens) are non-microbial, allergy and infection are linked in a number of ways. Most striking are the worm infections. As mentioned in the previous chapter, escape of antigen from a hydatid cyst can precipitate massive anaphylaxis—a dreaded complication of surgical removal of large cysts (Fig. 22.2). Roundworms like *Ascaris*, which sometimes visit the lung, can precipitate violent asthmatic attacks. Why worms are so prone to induce so much non-specific as well as specific IgE antibody is not understood, but there is evidence that specific IgE and eosinophils constitute a killing mechanism against some worms, so there may be some protective advantage. Some of the symptoms of respiratory virus infections may also be due to type I hypersensitivity, though it can be difficult to distinguish these from the effects of the virus itself (sneezing, mucus secretion, etc.). In addition, an upper respiratory virus infection may trigger allergy or asthma in an already atopic individual (e.g. to pollen).

Most interesting of all is the proposed link between childhood exposure to infectious disease and the later development of allergy—the *hygiene* hypothesis. According to this idea the increased level of allergic disease in developed countries is due to the later and lesser exposure to various pathogens, perhaps especially enteric organisms. The mechanism might operate via the T_H2/T_H1 axis or by a general effect of regulatory T (and other) cells secreting, for instance IL-10, in response to a range of infections. IL-10 has a 'damping down' effect on almost all immune responses, both innate and adaptive, and has been referred to as the 'homeostatic' cytokine. Another indirect link between infection and allergy is the unfortunate tendency of many *antibiotics* to induce allergic reactions—penicillin being the most obvious example (see Chapter 28 for further details).

Type II (cytotoxic) hypersensitivity

Here it is the ability of IgG antibody to destroy cells by causing them to be either phagocytosed or lysed by complement (IgM will do the latter too) that causes the trouble. Normally, of course, IgG is just what is wanted to get rid of pathogens, but in two special circumstances phagocytosis and lysis are not wanted. One is when removal of the cells is not desired, although they are foreign, obvious examples being a blood transfusion or a bone marrow graft. The other is when the IgG is directed against self; this is *autoimmunity*, an important complication of some infections, to be discussed in the following chapter. Sometimes included in this group, though not actually cytotoxic, are the cases where antibody against *hormone receptors* can bind to the receptor and either stimulate or inhibit it; thyroid diseases are the best-validated examples of this but there is no clear link to infection. However, some authorities prefer to call this type V hypersensitivity.

Type III (immune complex-mediated) hypersensitivity

Here, too, IgG antibody is involved, but the damage is actually initiated by soluble complexes of antigen and antibody. The antigen may be self (autoantibodies to DNA are particularly important in some chronic diseases) or of microbial origin. The damage is due to the fact that, though of course complexing with antigen for subsequent removal is the whole point of making antibody, large amounts of antigen–antibody complexes cannot always be removed from the blood rapidly enough, and tend to end up in the tissues or, more seriously, in the walls of small blood vessels. Here they can be attacked by the combination of PMNs and complement (both of which are involved in the protective effects of antibody, see Chapter 11 and Table 16.1). Under these conditions, PMNs may release their toxic contents and damage the blood vessel. Platelets also contribute to the damage. The skin and the renal glomerulus are two particularly vulnerable sites, but any small vessel can be affected. Prolonged immune complex deposition in the kidney is one of the commonest causes of *glomerulonephritis*, which in turn is the commonest cause of renal failure. Several infectious diseases are among the causes of glomerulonephritis (Table 22.3) and quite often an infectious organism is suspected but cannot be identified.

In the pre-penicillin days when injection of horse antibodies was the only treatment for bacterial pneumonia, etc., immune complexes formed between the horse immunoglobulins and human antibodies against them, deposited at several sites in the body, gave rise to the syndrome of *serum sickness*, with damage to skin, kidney, and joints; generally this got better when the injections were stopped. The modern use of 'humanized' monoclonal antibodies has eliminated this complication.

Table 22.3 Glomerulonephritis and other forms of vasculitis can be caused by immune complexes formed during the course of various infectious diseases. These would all be regarded as examples of type III hypersensitivity

Organ(s) affected	Infectious organism	Condition
Renal glomerulus	Hepatitis B virus	Chronic hepatitis
	Staphylococcus	Endocarditis
	Streptococcus	Post-streptococcal infection
	Treponema pallidum	Secondary syphilis
	Plasmodium	Malaria
	falciparum	malignant tertian
	malariae	quartan
	Schistosomes	Schistosomiasis
Other blood vessels (in skin, joints, etc.)	Hepatitis B	Acute hepatitis
	Mycobacterium leprae	Leprosy
	? Hepatitis B, ? TB	Polyarteritis nodosa
	Dengue virus	Haemorrhagic fever

Type IV (cell-mediated) hypersensitivity

This term refers to the harmful aspects of cell-mediated immune responses, the principal one being excessive *granuloma* formation. As explained in Chapter 19, the formation of a granuloma may sometimes be the best way to control an intracellular infection that even activated macrophages cannot totally eliminate; the solid mass of macrophages, fibrous tissue, etc. being an effective 'walling-off' device as well as providing enhanced killing potential. However, very numerous confluent granulomas can displace so much normal tissue that they interfere with normal function. Moreover, some of them tend to become necrotic at the centre. This combination of *fibrosis* and *cavitation* is a frequent end-result of pulmonary tuberculosis (Fig. 22.3). In some diseases (e.g. sarcoidosis) granulomas form but no microbial cause can be identified. In others, the organism is known, but not the mechanism. An example is *farmer's lung*, a serious hypersensitivity reaction to fungal spores (and some animal products) whose pathogenesis seems to include features of both type III and type IV.

Just as allergic status can be measured by an immediate skin test (see above), the level of cell-mediated hypersensitivity can be detected by a *delayed* skin test. For example, if an intradermal injection of purified protein antigens from the tubercle bacillus (PPD) encounters specific T helper cells, a local inflammatory reaction, with oedema and cellular infiltration, develops over the next 2–3 days—a

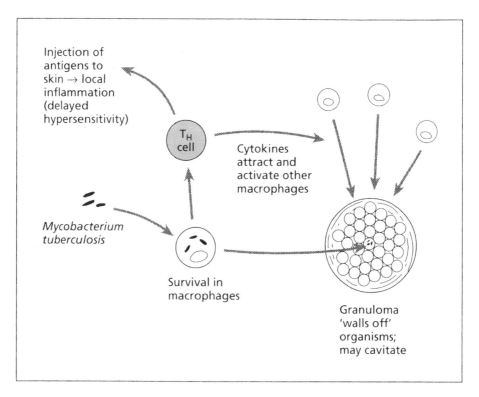

Fig. 22.3 Granuloma formation in tuberculosis, and the elicitation of a positive delayed (Mantoux) skin test, are both dependent on the existence of mycobacterial antigen specific T cells (CD4+, T_H1 type). Both phenomena are covered by the term type IV hypersensitivity. For further details see Fig. 19.3.

positive *delayed hypersensitivity* (DTH) test. DTH tests are often named in relation to the disease in question; thus Tuberculin (for TB), Lepromin (for leprosy), and leishmanin (for leishmaniasis). Note, however, that a positive Mantoux (tuberculin) test does not guarantee that the patient is 'immune' to TB, merely that there has been previous exposure, so that one cannot automatically equate delayed hypersensitivity with protection.

Another situation where cell-mediated reactions harm tissues is the killing of virus-infected cells by CTLs (see Fig. 19.4). On balance this is beneficial in disposing of the virus, but nevertheless there is damage to the host which can reach serious levels—as in the case of hepatitis and some respiratory viral infections. The damage to the liver in hepatitis B, which may occasionally be life-threatening, is mainly due to CTLs, since the virus itself is not cytopathic.

23 Disease due to adaptive immunity II: autoimmunity

In the previous chapter, several examples were given where damage to the host is due to an adaptive immune response against 'self' antigens. In some cases this can be traced to an infectious organism, but often the cause is unknown. Of the large number of possible reasons for *autoimmunity*, four can be identified as fairly well established:

(1) *polyclonal* activation of anti-self B or T lymphocytes;

(2) activation of auto-reactive B or T lymphocytes by antigens closely similar to self: *molecular mimicry*;

(3) release of *sequestered* antigens;

(4) anomalous *antigen presentation*.

Self-tolerance

Before discussing these further, we need to understand how autoimmunity is normally avoided (Fig. 23.1). Why do some B and T lymphocytes not recognize and respond to 'self' antigens, considering that their receptors are produced by a random recombination of genes and should be able to recognize virtually everything, instead of being unresponsive, or *tolerant*, to self? The explanation is different for B and T cells. In the case of B cells, many self-reactive cells do in fact exist, though probably those with really high affinity for self antigens are eliminated in the bone marrow. T cells, however, are 'vetted' much more scrupulously: by means of a two-stage selection process in the thymus, the great majority of those that recognize *self MHC plus a self peptide* are eliminated. This means that few or no T cells will respond to *unaltered* self, and therefore a B cell, even if it does recognize a self antigen, will generally not get help from a T cell: it is 'anergic'. This ensures that only low-affinity IgM antibody is normally made against self antigens, and only those of the 'repeating epitope' kind (see Fig. 18.2). There are also thought to be mechanisms for rendering T cells anergic in the periphery, under the influence of special 'tolerogenic' dendritic cells or of regulatory T cells.

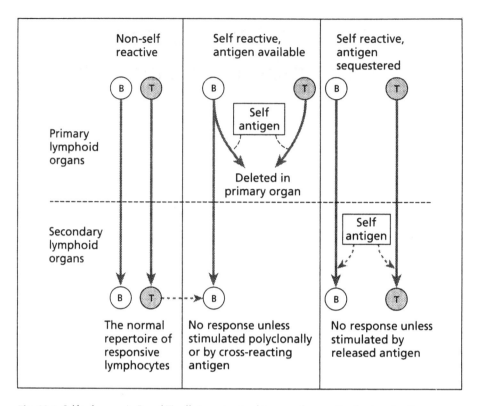

Fig. 23.1 Self-tolerance in B and T cells is maintained in several ways. For further details, see text.

Polyclonal lymphocyte activation

This embargo on responses by self-reactive B cells, however, can be broken by molecules with the property of triggering responses by all, or a high proportion of, lymphocytes. In the case of B cells, many such molecules are of plant origin, but they also include molecules from bacteria such as LPS, from protozoa—notably malaria and trypanosomes—and viruses such as EBV and hepatitis C. Infections of all these kinds are accompanied by high levels of IgM antibody, most of which is not directed at the microbial antigens, but some of which may be directed against self. Usually this is not serious, and the autoantibodies disappear when (and if) the infection is cleared. But it has been suggested that in some diseases associated with IgG autoantibodies (for example systemic lupus erythematosus and rheumatoid arthritis), the above process has got out of control (Fig. 23.2). Possibly in these cases the T cells are being activated by *superantigens* from bacteria or viruses (see Chapter 17), though at present it is thought that these are more important in exacerbating already activated autoimmunity than in initiating it.

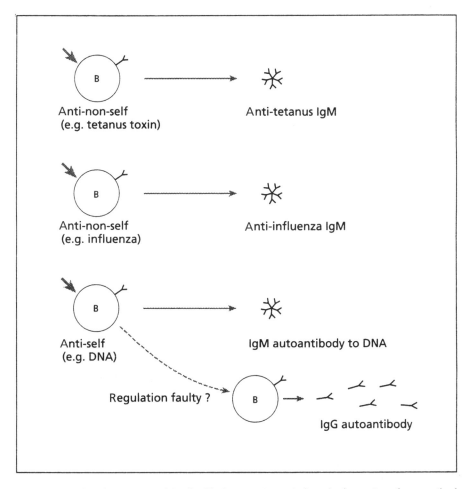

Fig. 23.2 Polyclonal activation of B cells (black arrows) may induce the formation of autoantibody by any self-reactive cells that have escaped elimination in the bone marrow.

Antigen mimicry

Another way round the absence of self-reactive T cells is for an antigen to carry both 'self' and 'non-self' determinants, thus partially *mimicking* its host and 'by-passing' the lack of self-reactive T cells. Provided a B cell can recognize the self portion and a T cell the non-self portion, the T cell will supply help, resulting in a full-blown antibody response to the self portion. An example is the group A streptococcus, which happens to carry an antigen very similar to one on mammalian heart muscle, kidney, and joints. Antibodies to this antigen can therefore damage these organs, and this explains the myocarditis seen in rheumatic fever. Figure 23.3 illustrates this mechanism and Table 23.1 lists some other examples of molecular mimicry by microbes. Another way of arriving at the same result is

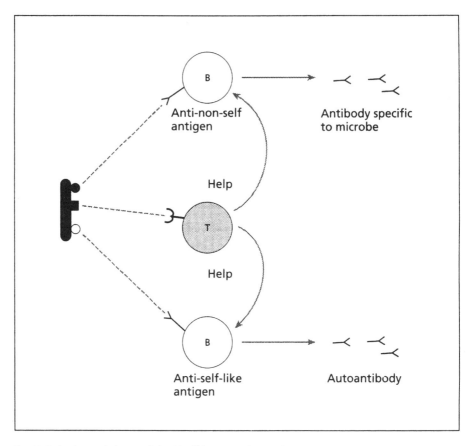

Fig. 23.3 Antigen mimicry and the 'T-cell bypass'. The combination of foreign (*solid circles*) and self (*open circles*) antigens on a microbe allows a T-dependent autoantibody response, bypassing the lack of self-reactive T helper cells.

for a foreign molecule to bind to a host cell and supply a 'carrier' antigen for normal T cells to recognize; this is thought to be what happens when penicillin, which binds to red cells, causes an autoimmune haemolytic anaemia.

Molecular mimicry can also operate at the T cell level, because MHC-peptide binding (see above) is *degenerate*—that is, one MHC molecule can bind more than one peptide, provided certain critical amino acid residues are present. Thus a microbial peptide could be similar enough to a self-peptide to trigger T cells which can go on to respond to unaltered self (one can imagine that if *all* T cells were deleted that recognized 'near-self', very few would be left to cope with non-self!). Once one self peptide has been recognized, others on the same molecule may be drawn in—the concept of *epitope spreading*. Many examples have been found in animal experiments. One group of antigens that display great similarity between microbe and host are the *heat shock proteins* released during tissue

Table 23.1 Some examples of molecular mimicry between pathogens and their hosts. For those asterisked, there is reasonable evidence that they are involved in the induction of autoimmunity

Viruses
Vaccinia	IL-1 receptor
Epstein–Barr	IL-10
Cytomegalovirus	β2 microglobulin; chemokine receptor
Herpes simplex	Complement receptor 1
Polio	Acetylcholine receptor
Hepatitis B	Myelin basic protein
Rabies	Insulin receptor
Adenovirus	*α gliadin (a wheat component)
Herpes (monkey)	IL-8 receptor
Sarcoma viruses (cat, mouse, etc.)	Host oncogenes

Bacteria
Group A streptococci	*Human myocardial myosin
Klebsiella	*HLA B 27
Meningococcus	Fetal brain
Treponema (syphilis)	*Cardiolipin (a phospholipid)
Mycoplasma	*Blood group I antigen
Campylobacter jejuni	*Peripheral nerve gangliosides

Fungi
Candida	Complement receptor 3

Protozoa
Plasmodium (malaria)	Thymus hormone
Trypanosoma cruzi	Human heart and nerve antigens

Worms
Schistosoma	Glutathione transferase

damage and able to activate CD8 T cells as well as many innate immune mechanisms.

Mimicry of the streptococcal kind is sometimes cited as an example of pathogens trying to escape the immune system, but whether it actually contributes to this is debatable. There are many much more effective escape mechanisms open to the pathogen. On the other hand, the mimicry of cytokines and signalling molecules by viruses may be a major element in pathogen survival (see Chapter 21).

Release of sequestered antigens

Whatever the mechanism of tolerance, if B and T lymphocytes do not meet a self antigen, they cannot develop tolerance to it. This is particularly the case with lens and sperm proteins. Thus if the corresponding organ is damaged, the lymphocytes will see the antigens as foreign and mount an immune response. This can happen in the testis during mumps, and accounts for a small proportion of male sterility (see Fig. 23.1).

Anomalous antigen presentation

One of the striking findings in organs affected by autoimmunity—for example the thyroid and the pancreatic islets—is the appearance of MHC class II antigens on cells where they are normally absent. It is thought that this may be due to local production of cytokines, especially IFNγ, perhaps in response to virus infection. One result might be that thyroid or islet cells can now present antigens to T cells, including their own surface or secreted molecules, which in turn would allow B cells to make antibodies against them (Fig. 23.4). Another possibility would be that the pathogen increases costimulatory activity; the experimental use of mycobacteria as *adjuvants* for autoimmunity may be an example of this. This whole concept still requires firm proof, but it illustrates another way in which infection might lead indirectly to autoimmunity.

Autoimmunity, autoimmune disease, and genetics

Finally, it should be stressed that the presence of *autoantibodies* does not automatically lead to disease, and in fact it has only been proved for a few diseases that they are actually caused by the autoantibodies rather than vice versa; these include thyrotoxicosis, myasthenia gravis, and the skin disease pemphigus. Others, such as diabetes, may be largely T-cell-mediated, while others, such as haemolytic anaemia, can be due to normal immune responses against foreign antigens that happen to bind to self cells—in this case red cells (see above).

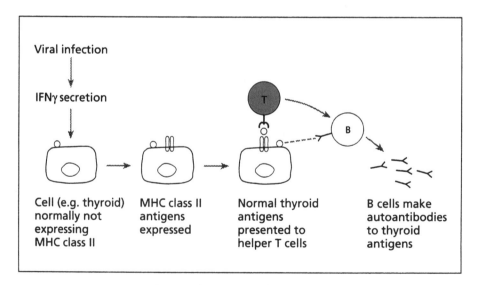

Fig. 23.4 The 'anomalous MHC expression' hypothesis for autoimmunity. Note that the abnormal MHC expression could also be secondary, i.e. due to cytokines produced during an already established autoimmune thyroiditis.

A striking feature of almost all autoimmune diseases is the predominance of particular HLA types. In one group of rheumatological diseases, headed by ankylosing spondylitis, the association is with B27, possibly because of mimicry of this molecule by bacterial antigens. A range of other autoimmune diseases is more weakly associated with the combination B8 DR3, and here the suspicion is that the control of cytokine responses is defective. There may also be defects in genes such as Fas, required for T cell deletion. Interestingly, autoimmune diseases in general are less common in tropical countries, perhaps due to a protective effect by protozoal or worm infections.

24 Immunodeficiency II: primary defects of adaptive immunity

First, look back at Chapter 14 to be reminded about the difference between primary (genetic) and secondary (acquired) immunodeficiency. As you will see from Fig. 14.1, primary immunodeficiencies affecting the adaptive immune system—that is, *lymphocyte* function—are about five times commoner than those affecting innate immunity (complement, phagocytes, etc.), which were discussed in Chapter 14. Note, however, that in terms of total incidence, secondary immunodeficiencies (see Chapter 25) considerably outnumber them both.

Just as with the innate defects, primary adaptive immunodeficiencies are inherited, so that they are either X-linked or autosomal. Depending on the nature of the defect, it may show up at an early or a late stage of lymphocyte differentiation, affecting T cells, B cells (i.e. antibody), or both (Fig. 24.1). Of course, since much antibody formation depends on healthy T cells, a pure T cell defect may present with an antibody problem too. Generally the defect becomes evident because of repeated or unusual infections or a failure to respond to vaccination. Diagnosis, formerly based on the clinical condition, can nowadays usually be made with great precision by identifying the abnormal or missing gene.

Defects affecting T and B cells

Defects that act at the earliest precursor stages in the bone marrow, or on some function vital to both types of cell, will show up as a combination of T and B cell deficiency.

(1) *Reticular dysgenesis*. A bone-marrow stem-cell failure, incompatible with survival.

(2) *Ataxia telangectasia*. A defect in the normal mechanism by which damaged DNA is repaired, with multiple consequences, both to the immune system (hypoplastic thymus, IgA deficiency) and elsewhere (brain, liver, skin).

(3) *Wiskott–Aldrich syndrome*. An X-linked combination of defects at the level of platelets (bleeding), skin (eczema), and antibody formation to polysaccharides (infection with capsulated bacteria). The defect is in the WASP protein responsible for cytoskeletal function, required for normal cell morphology, movement, and adhesion—including T–B cell interaction.

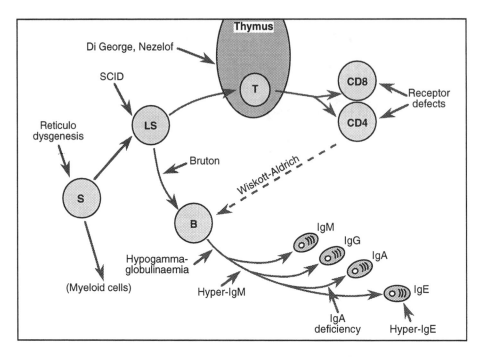

Fig. 24.1 A simplified scheme of haemopoiesis, showing the site of the defect in the major lymphoid immunodeficiencies. S: bone marrow stem cell; LS: lymphoid stem cell; T: T lymphocyte; B: B lymphocyte. SCID: Severe combined immunodeficiency.

(4) *Severe combined immunodeficiency (SCID).* A heterogeneous group of defects at the level of lymphocyte precursors. The common feature is a severe reduction or absence of T cells, with variable reductions in B cells. There are two main types: (1) a lesion in enzymes of the purine pathway, either adenosine deaminase (ADA) or purine nucleoside phosphorylase (PNP), allowing a build-up of dATP or dGTP which are toxic to lymphoid stem cells; (2) an X-linked defect in a common cytokine receptor chain, required for the maturation of lymphoid stem cells. Treatment of SCID deficiency by gene therapy has been tried (see later).

Defects affecting T cells

(1) *Di George syndrome.* A failure of embryonic development of the 3rd and 4th pharyngeal pouches, resulting in absence of the thymus and parathyroids, with facial and cardiac abnormalities. Cases usually present rapidly with tetany due to the lack of parathyroid hormone; the immunological defect was originally noticed when affected babies developed massive vaccinia infections following the smallpox vaccine and on X-ray the thymus shadow was seen to be missing. Treatment with fetal thymus grafting has shown

some success, but spontaneous improvement may occur due to compensatory non-thymic development of T cells.

(2) *Nezelof syndrome*. Somewhat similar to the above, but with normal parathyroids.

(3) *PNP deficiency* (see above) may affect only T cell development.

(4) *T-cell receptor (TCR) defects*. Lesions can occur in the recombinase genes necessary for the proper rearrangement of germ-line V, D, and J segments into a functional TCR, resulting in an absence of TCR and failure of T cells to be activated. Defects in TCR-associated signalling molecules such as ZAP-70 will have the same effect.

(5) *MHC and antigen presentation defects*. There may be absence or low levels of MHC molecules, or defects in the processes by which they pick up and transport antigen within the antigen-presenting cells. In the *bare lymphocyte syndrome* there is an absence of both HLA class I and class II.

Defects affecting B cells and antibody

(1) *Agammaglobulinaemia* (Bruton's disease). An X-linked absence of B cells and thus of immunoglobulin, caused by a number of different mutations in the tyrosine kinase gene. There may also be intermittent reductions in neutrophils. Patients typically present with pyogenic infections. The disease was first spotted in 1952 in a boy with recurrent pneumonia, thanks to the newly invented immunoelectrophoresis technique for demonstrating immunoglobulins in the serum (Fig. 24.2).

(2) *Hypogammaglobulinaemia*. More commonly, low levels of IgG or IgA are found, often with normal numbers of B cells in the bone marrow, but a failure to develop properly into plasma cells. The heterogeneous nature of this group of defects is reflected in the name *common variable immunodeficiency*.

(3) *Selective IgA deficiency* is remarkable in being quite common (about 1 in 800 Caucasians) and often symptomless.

(4) *X-linked hyper-IgM syndromes*. Two T cell defects have their effect on the B-cell IgM–IgG switch. (1) Caused by a mutation in the gene for the CD40 ligand, which is involved in the switch from IgM to IgG, etc. and also T cell–macrophage interaction. As a result there are raised levels of IgM and reduced levels of IgG and IgA, an absence of germinal centres and somatic hypermutation, and sometimes defects in cell-mediated immunity. (2) Caused by a mutation in an enzyme, AID, leading to giant germinal centres.

(5) *Hyper-IgE syndrome (Job syndrome)*. Characterized by raised serum IgE and repeated skin infections.

(6) Recombinase defects, as with T cells.

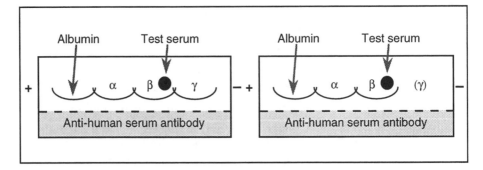

Fig. 24.2 Immunoelectrophoresis of (left) normal and (right) agammaglobulinaemic serum. Note the absence of the precipitation arc corresponding to the gammaglobulins.

Clinical aspects of primary immune deficiencies

Though they are rare, primary immune deficiencies represent one of the best opportunities for immunological principles to be applied to human disease (another, *vaccination*, was established long before anything was known about immunology). Infant lives which would certainly have been lost until a few decades ago are now regularly being saved, chiefly in specialist centres where diagnosis and treatment can be carried out.

Diagnosis

Severe recurrent infections in a young child should always alert the doctor to the possibility of a primary immune deficiency, particularly if the infection is an unusual one. To some extent the nature of the infection will suggest where the defect is (see Table 25.7 in the following chapter for a summary). Note that, because of the cooperation of antibody, complement, and phagocytic cells, defects of any of these predispose to much the same range of infections.

Routine tests exist for measuring blood T cell, B cell, NK cell, and myeloid cell numbers, using flow cytometry and monoclonal antibodies against specific cell-surface markers (e.g. CD3, 4, and 8 for T cells, T_H cells, and T_C cells, respectively). Serum antibody levels are easily measured using ELISA. T and B cell function can be broadly assessed by their proliferative and cytokine response on culture with various mitogens (e.g. PHA for T cells) or specific 'recall' antigens. The oxygen burst in neutrophils (e.g. for chronic granulomatous disease) can be checked with the NBT test—a simple rapid colour change. Where a particular gene defect is suspected, Northern blotting (for mRNA) or gene sequencing (for DNA) can be applied. Though there will undoubtedly be improvements, these kinds of test can usually indicate whether there is a significant immune defect or not. Unfortunately there remain patients with clearly increased susceptibility to, for example, upper respiratory viruses or skin infections, in whom no obvious defect can be traced. In fact the extent to which *minor ill-health* has an immunological basis remains a field that has hardly been explored.

Treatment

Treatment of an immunodeficient patient can be directed (1) at reducing their infection(s), and/or (2) replacing the defect.

Reducing infection

Obviously avoiding likely sources of infection makes sense; for example a patient with a T cell deficiency should not come in contact with cases of TB or be given a live viral vaccine. Very severe immunodeficiency may require complete isolation—a very distressing and expensive process. For infections with identified organisms, chemotherapy is the mainstay—antibacterial, antifungal, etc. as appropriate (see Chapter 28). Some conditions respond to cytokines, the best example being the effect of repeated injections of IFNγ in some cases of CGD.

Replacement therapy

Most patients with hypogammaglobulinaemia can be kept healthy by monthly injections of pooled normal human immunoglobulin. This is a vivid demonstration that normal people have protective levels of antibody against common pathogens. Another, perhaps surprising, form of replacement therapy is the transfusion of normal red blood cells for ADA deficiency, but of course neither of these non-self-renewing treatments constitutes a cure. For this it is necessary to permanently replace the defective *cell* or *gene*.

Bone marrow transplantation

All the cellular components of the immune system are derived ultimately from the bone marrow, so a successful graft of normal marrow should theoretically be

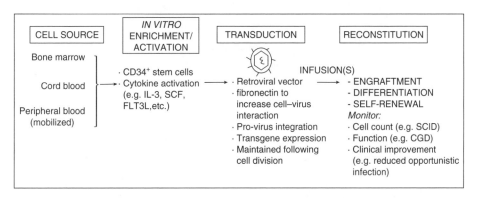

Fig. 24.3 The major approaches to gene therapy of immune deficiencies. SCF: Stem cell factor; FLT3L: FLT3 ligand.

able to replace any of them. In practice, because of its dangers (see below) this is reserved for severe cases, notably SCID; nearly 400 successful treatments of this condition have been carried out worldwide to date. A good HLA match between host and donor is desirable, not so much to avoid rejection (the patients are already immunodeficient!) but to prevent *graft-versus-host* (GVH) disease. This is the situation where the injected marrow attempts to reject the host, causing severe damage to epithelial cells in the gut, liver, and skin, which is frequently fatal. It is minimized by (a) ensuring the best possible HLA match; (b) depletion of T cells from the marrow before grafting—where possible only those with potential reactivity against host HLA; (c) the administration of the cytokine GM-CSF; and (d) on an experimental basis, the use of purified stem cells.

Gene therapy

This is the most logical approach, since most primary defects are of a single gene, and even a partial restoration of levels of the missing protein may be quite beneficial. Being still experimental, this technique is reserved for life-threatening conditions, particularly SCID. A normal version of the defective gene can be inserted into the patient's own T cells or, better, stem cells, using a suitable retrovirus, modified so as not to be pathogenic (Fig. 24.3). The major problems so far are (1) the rather low efficiency of gene insertion, and (2) the inability to control where the new gene is inserted; one would not want it to go into a site where it could disturb normal cell growth control. Recent (2003) cases of leukaemia in treated children are a hint that this problem may be a real one.

25 Immunodeficiency III: secondary immunodeficiency and AIDS

In contrast to the inborn primary immunodeficiencies already described, secondary immunodeficiency results from some influence *external* to the immune system—infection, malnutrition, etc. (see below)—ranging from the slightly increased risk of infection following surgery to the severe and progressive immune failure of HIV/AIDS. Most adult immunodeficiency falls into this category, and since both innate and adaptive immunity can be affected, they will be discussed together here. In fact the defects in secondary immunodeficiencies are usually multiple and complex, so that the only effective treatment is to remove the external cause, if possible. The principal causes are listed in Table 25.1. Note that several forms of medical treatment can themselves cause *iatrogenic* immunodeficiency.

Malnutrition

When either total calorie or protein intake falls below a certain level, antibody production is severely affected and, to a lesser extent, complement levels, and phagocytes. There may also be atrophy of lymphoid tissues, especially the thymus, and loss of T cell function. This is probably the main reason why infections normally regarded as minor, such as measles, can be so severe in the tropics, the complications including pneumonia, otitis, diarrhoea, and massive haemorrhagic rashes. It is estimated that a million children die per year from measles worldwide. A normal intake of iron (see below) and zinc is also necessary for healthy immunity, and the effects of these and other food supplements including vitamins on chronic infection and in the elderly are currently being tested. Interestingly, a few diseases (e.g. typhus) appear to be *less* severe in malnourished patients, and here one would suspect that the symptoms may themselves be immunological in nature (see Chapter 22). Note that malnutrition may itself be secondary to renal failure, drug therapy, etc.

Iron

Iron metabolism is strictly controlled and either deficiency or excess can increase susceptibility to infection (see Table 25.2). On the one hand iron is a key

Table 25.1 The commonest causes of secondary immunodeficiency

Condition	Main causes	Major elements affected
Malnutrition	Protein-energy, iron, zinc deficiency	Antibody
Infection	HIV, CMV, EBV, measles, TB, leprosy, brucella, syphilis, malaria, sleeping sickness	T cells
Tumours	Lymphoid: myeloma, CLL, Hodgkin's, NHL, other	Multiple
Trauma	Burns, wounds, surgery, Splenectomy	Cytokines, monocytes Clearance from blood
Medical treatment	Drugs: steroids, Imuran, Cyclophosphamide, X-irradiation	Neutrophils
Protein loss	Diarrhoea, nephrotic syndrome, burns	Multiple
Other	Diabetes, renal failure, haemochromatosis	Multiple

CMV, cytomegalovirus; EBV, Epstein–Barr virus; CLL, chronic lymphoid leukaemia; NHL, non-Hodgkin's lymphoma.

Table 25.2 The balance between iron deficiency and overload

Iron deficiency	Iron overload
Dietary	Haemochromatosis (see below)
Blood loss	Dietary
	Chronic hepatitis C
	Blood transfusion
	Thalassaemia

cofactor of many host enzymes involved in immune function, particularly the reactive oxygen intermediates responsible for killing of pathogens in neutrophils. On the other hand many bacteria, fungi, and protozoa require adequate concentrations of iron for their own growth, and some have multiple siderophores which scavenge iron from the environment. There is thus a competitive battle for iron between host and pathogen. In malaria, iron deficiency may actually reduce the severity of infection because of the parasite's need for healthy red cells to grow in, and there is also the special case of sickle-cell anaemia, in which heterozygotes for the abnormal haemoglobin HbS are relatively resistant to *Plasmodium falciparum*. Some cytokines (e.g. IFNγ, TNF) can decrease the available iron pool by raising the level of the iron-binding protein ferritin. Neutrophil-derived lactoferrin has the same effect.

Iron overload is seen in several situations (see Table 25.2) and can have deleterious effects on the function of macrophages, neutrophils, NK cells, and lymphocytes.

Infection

The ability of some infections to cause immunodeficiency, thus predisposing the patient to other infections, is of great interest and importance, and the AIDS epidemic has brought home to the developed world the way in which infectious organisms can interact with one another in the same host. A successful treatment for AIDS (e.g. HAART, see below) if globally available, would relegate such organisms as *Pneumocystis carinii*, currently a major cause of death in AIDS patients (and the clue that led, in 1981, to the first description of the disease) to the small print of microbiology textbooks where it previously languished.

HIV and AIDS

The human immunodeficiency viruses HIV-1 and -2 are unique in that their primary target of attack is the cells of the immune system, which they progressively damage to the point where the patient succumbs, usually to another infection. The reason the immune system is singled out is that HIV uses as its cell receptor the CD4 molecule (see Chapter 17 and Fig. 17.4), which is found mainly on T helper cells, dendritic cells, and macrophages, but also on some other cells including parts of the brain. Entry also requires a second receptor—one of two molecules, CCR5 and CXCR4, whose normal function is to act as receptors for chemokines (see Chapter 11). One of the viral surface antigens, known as gp (glycoprotein) 120, binds to these receptors and allows the virus to enter and multiply, predominantly in lymph nodes, spreading from cell to cell by budding. The requirement for the CD4 molecule means that only T cells and antigen-presenting cells are affected, so that some immune responses, e.g. antibody, remain fairly normal. Moreover some immunopathological consequences of infection may actually be reduced—for example the systemic spread of candida and the formation of cavities in TB.

Spread to a new host can occur by sexual contact, contaminated blood, or from mother to newborn. It was originally assumed that infection with HIV simply destroyed helper T cells, but it is almost certainly not as simple as this, and a number of other possible mechanisms have been proposed (Table 25.3). Even in advanced disease, not more than about 1 per cent of CD4 T cells in the blood actually contain the virus, although the numbers are much higher in lymph nodes where the virus replicates.

HIV-1 and -2 are retroviruses (see Fig. 2.2), and contain a number of unusual

Table 25.3 Numerous theories have been advanced to explain why HIV, without infecting all T helper cells, causes a progressive loss of their numbers and function

---

Direct effects on T cells
    *Lysis by HIV (infected cells only)
    *Suppressed production, thymic failure
    *Persistent immune overactivation, clonal expansion, death

Lysis by CD8 cytotoxic cells (infected cells, and cells binding HIV antigens)
    Fusion (syncytium formation) and death
    Selective loss of memory cells;* apoptosis

Immunosuppression
    By free gp 120 molecules blocking CD4 function
    By T_H2 cytokines (IL-4, IL-10) inhibiting protective T_H1 responses
    *Of antigen-presenting cell function by loss of follicular dendritic cells

Autoimmunity
    To CD4 or other T cell antigens
    To uninfected cells binding HIV antigen
    To self-MHC due to cross-reaction with HIV

---

* Currently most favoured.

Table 25.4 HIV genes and their function

Gene	Function encoded
5'LTR	(long terminal repeat) promoter, enhancer, DNA integrating
gag	core proteins p24, p17, p7
pol	(polymerase) reverse transcriptase, protease, integrase, RNAase
vif	viral infectivity factor
vpr	weak transcriptional factor, etc.
tat	transactivator; replication protein
rev	regulator virion proteins
vpu	virion budding, reduced CD4 expression
env	gp160 (cleaved to gp120, gp41) envelope proteins
nef	negative regulatory factor, reduced CD4 and MHC expression
3'LTR	links to 5'LTR

genes that help to control their replication and integration into host DNA (Table 25.4). They are closely related to two African animal immunodeficiency viruses; HIV-1 is thought to have reached humans from chimpanzees and the less frequent HIV-2 from the SIV of sooty mangabey monkeys. Both monkeys and chimpanzees appear to be able to maintain their T cell levels despite persistent infection, and do not develop AIDS—perhaps because of *less* vigorous general immune activation.

An important feature is that HIV, and especially gp 120, contains five *hyper-variable regions*, V1–5, remarkably subject to antigenic variation, especially V3, (at least 20 times more than influenza), both between patients and within a single individual. Both antibody and cytotoxic T cells are therefore only transiently effective. This is unfortunate because gp 120 would otherwise be an ideal molecule on which to base a vaccine. Thus HIV poses the same problem as influenza but much worse, and despite intensive research no obvious vaccine strategy has yet emerged. Anti-viral drugs were also not as successful as was originally hoped (see Chapter 28) and treatments aimed at stimulating immune function, for example administration of cytokines such as IL-2, have been fairly disappointing. However, a combination of three or more drugs, aimed at different targets—so-called Highly Active Anti-Retroviral Therapy or HAART—is proving effective (Table 25.5). Paradoxically, patients treated in this way may undergo severe tissue reactions caused by their recovering T cells responding to their opportunists—'immune reconstitution disease'.

Table 25.5 Combined therapy for AIDS

Class	Examples	Function
Nucleoside analogues	*AZT; *3TC; ddI; D4T; 1592U	Inhibit reverse transcriptase
Protease inhibitors	*Indinavir; ritonavir; saquinavir	Inhibit protease

* These three drugs are often used together—'triple therapy'.

The classic course of HIV infection includes four distinguishable stages (Table 25.6) with a rough average of 10 years between the initial infection and fully developed AIDS. However, it is now evident that not all infected individuals progress at the same rate (the disease was only recognized in 1981) and it is widely believed that other factors contribute to the final outcome. These may include other viruses and microorganisms, MHC type, age, nutrition, and possibly the precise strain of HIV contracted. Encouragingly, a small number of patients known to have been infected at least 13 years ago are still perfectly well, probably because they lack the 'second receptor' CCR5. Nevertheless, the steady increase in numbers—perhaps 50–60 million people infected and almost 20 million deaths—and the impact of HIV on a disease like tuberculosis, which was hitherto thought to be coming under control but is now ravaging tropical countries, make HIV the most feared of all infectious organisms and a huge challenge to everyone concerned with infectious disease at any level. The theory that AIDS is not caused by HIV at all is not nowadays taken seriously.

Table 25.6 Infection with HIV normally leads to a steady progression of symptoms as the number of CD4 T cells falls, but some features (*) are not always seen. For a list of the common opportunist infections, see Table 25.7

Stage	Main symptoms	Blood tests		
		HIV antigen	Antibodies to HIV	CD4 T cells/µl
Acute	*Glandular fever-like illness	+ ↓ −	− ↓ +	1000
*Progressive generalized lymphadenopathy	Enlarged lymph nodes	−	+	
*AIDS-related complex (ARC)	Weight loss, fever, diarrhoea, opportunist infections	−	+	*c.* 500
AIDS	Kaposi's sarcoma Lymphomas Major opportunist infections *Encephalopathy, neuropathy *Dementia	+	+	200 or less

Other infections

No other infection has such a disastrous effect on the immune system as HIV, but the immunosuppression caused by the other infections listed in Table 25.1 can be quite serious. For example quite mild malaria can impair the response to pneumococcal and meningococcal vaccines, as was demonstrated in Nigeria by giving a course of antimalarial therapy before vaccination. Polyclonal activation of lymphocytes (e.g. of B cells by EB virus, malaria, leprosy, and T cells by staphylococcal superantigens) no doubt contributes to the immunosuppression seen in these diseases, though whether this benefits the pathogen is hard to establish. Measles, by infecting T lymphocytes and antigen presenting cells, suppresses cell-mediated immunity and can cause tuberculosis to flare up. The way in which herpes viruses interfere with the cytokine network has been mentioned in Chapters 12 and 21, and in this case it seems likely that the immunosuppression does have a survival advantage to these very persistent pathogens.

Other causes of immunodeficiency

Tumours

Space-occupying tumours growing in the bone marrow (e.g. leukaemia, myeloma, metastases) can directly inhibit leucocyte production. Others (e.g. Hodgkin's lymphoma) can do the same by secreting inhibitory cytokines. Remember also that anti-cancer therapy, whether irradiation or chemotherapy, will inhibit the production of all actively dividing cells, including immunological ones, the effect being most rapid and severe on short-lived cells such as polymorphs.

Trauma and sepsis

The systemic inflammatory (shock) reaction following massive endotoxin release in Gram-negative sepsis has been mentioned in Chapter 13. In survivors, this may be followed by a stage of overcompensation during which inflammatory and immune responses are damped down and susceptibility to other infections increased. A similar phenomenon can occur after major trauma, blood loss, burning, and even post-operatively (Fig. 25.1). The exact mechanisms are unclear but may include the production of inhibitory cytokines such as IL-10 and

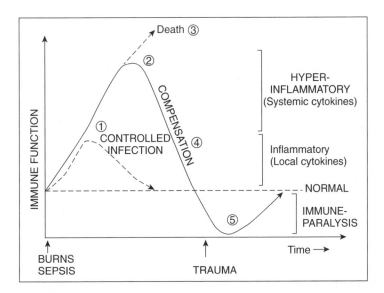

Fig. 25.1 The possible effects on the immune system of septic or post-traumatic shock (1) control of infection, with local cytokine production and transient inflammation; (2) hyper-inflammatory reaction with systemic cytokine levels, which may lead to either (3) death or (4) compensatory anti-inflammatory control mechanisms; (5) immune paralysis.

TGFβ, and treatments such as plasmapheresis (to remove inhibitory molecules) or the administration of stimulatory cytokines are being considered.

Splenectomy carries the special risk of infection with capsulated bacteria (and the otherwise harmless protozoal parasite *Babesia*), which are normally cleared by this organ. Splenectomized patients are generally vaccinated against *S. pneumoniae* as a precautionary measure.

Medical treatment

In addition to chemotherapy for cancer, a number of deliberately immunosuppressive drugs are used to reduce inflammation and various immunopathological conditions. A list of these is given in Table 20.1. Inevitably they carry with them the risk of infection.

Protein loss

In conditions of increased glomerular permeability (the nephrotic syndrome), in addition to albumin, immunoglobulins and complement components may be lost into the urine, resulting in an increased susceptibility to bacterial infection.

Diabetes

Skin, soft tissue, and bone infections are well-known complications of diabetes. The main lesion is a failure of neutrophils and monocytes to increase their background level of anti-microbial activity (motility, phagocytosis, intracellular killing), and may be partly related to the raised blood sugar itself. Infections of the extremities are particularly common, and combined with the effects of the disease on small blood vessels, may lead to necrosis and gangrene, sometimes requring amputation.

Renal failure

Most cellular elements, but especially neutrophils, may be impaired in chronic renal failure, resulting in an increased risk of bacterial sepsis and poor responses to vaccination—particularly important in renal dialysis patients who have a higher risk of exposure to hepatitis viruses. Renal transplantation, with its associated immunosuppressive regime, will of course exacerbate the danger of infection.

Haemochromatosis

In this condition of iron overload, which may be primary (due to a mutation in the HLA-related Hfe gene) or secondary to overconsumption of iron, repeated blood transfusion, and haemolytic anaemias, bacterial and fungal infections are common (see above for a discussion of iron balance).

Immunity in the elderly

As the production of new T cells declines and existing cells near the end of their proliferative lifespan, the population is increasingly composed of memory cells. B cells, and cell–cell interaction, are also progressively impaired. Tuberculosis, pneumonia, urinary infection, and reactivation of herpesviruses (e.g. zoster) are commoner with age, and so is autoimmunity. However, studies on centenarians have shown remarkably normal levels of general immune competence.

Infections in the immunodeficient patient

Whatever the cause of the immunodeficiency, the resulting pattern of infection depends on the component affected; indeed from a knowledge of immunology one can more or less predict it. Broadly speaking, defects of phagocytes, comple-

Table 25.7 The major infections encountered in immunodeficient patients fall into two main sets: (*top*) those depending on antibody, complement, and phagocytes for their control and (*bottom*) those depending mainly on T cell-mediated responses. Note the importance of fungal infections in both groups

Deficiency	Major infections expected			
	Viruses	Bacteria	Fungi	Protozoa and worms
Phagocytes		*Staphylococcus* *Streptococcus* *Pseudomonas*	*Candida* *Aspergillus*	
CGD splenectomy		granulomata *Pneumococcus* *Meningococcus*		*Babesia*
Complement		*Staphylococcus* *Streptococcus* *Pseudomonas*		
lytic pathway		*Neisseria*		
Antibody	Enteroviruses	*Staphylococcus* *Streptococcus* *Haemophilus* *Pneumococcus*	*Pneumocystis*	*Giardia*
T cells	CMV, HSV EBV	*Listeria* *M. tuberculosis* *M leprae* Mycoplasma	*Candida* *Aspergillus* *Histoplasma* *Pneumocystis* *Cryptococcus*	*Strongyloides*
AIDS	CMV, HSV EBV HHV8	Mycobacteria (including *M. avium*)	*Cryptococcus* *Candida* *Pneumocystis*	*Cryptosporidium* *Toxoplasma*

CMV, cytomegalovirus; EBV, Epstein–Barr virus; HSV, herpes simplex virus; HHV, human herpes virus.

ment, or antibody predispose to infections with extracellular organisms, especially bacteria and fungi, and T cell defects to intracellular infections, including most viruses but also several important bacteria, fungi, and protozoa (see Table 25.7 and refer back to Chapters 14 and 24 for more details).

Treatment of secondary immunodeficiency

The mainstay of treatment is to treat the infection, and if possible the original cause. On a worldwide scale, *malnutrition* is by far the most common of these, which is particularly disastrous for tropical countries since they are also exposed to a much wider range of infectious organisms, many of which (e.g. most protozoa and worms) are restricted to these areas. The effect of adequate nutrition (and clean water) on the incidence of infection in the tropical world would probably outweigh the effects of all the vaccines and antibiotics in existence.

Tutorial 3

For many people this will be the most difficult part of the book, the activities of lymphocytes being so unlike those of any other type of cell. By attempting the following essays, you will discover where your weak spots (if any) lie, and which chapters may need going over again, supplemented by some further reading from the list on p. 301.

1. 'I assume . . . that all antibody molecules contain the same polypeptide chains . . . the antigen causes the polypeptide chains to assume a configuration complementary to the antigen.' (Pauling 1940)

   '. . . in the animal there exist clones of (lymphocytes) each carrying immunologically reactive sites corresponding . . . to one potential antigenic determinant . . . When an antigen is introduced it will make contact with a cell of the corresponding clone . . . and stimulate it to produce more globulin molecules of the cell's characteristic type.' (Burnet 1959)

   How do we know Burnet was right and Pauling wrong?

2. Why does an individual B cell retain only one out of hundreds of heavy chain V genes but a full set of C genes?

3. Without T cells, there would be no need for MHC molecules. Discuss.

4. Any successful parasite must be able to vary its antigens. Discuss.

5. The development of *memory* is the hallmark of the lymphocyte. Is it?

6. If a pathogen is to be eliminated, some damage to host tissues is inevitable. Is it?

7. An 8-year-old boy who had recovered normally from chickenpox 4 years earlier but suffered repeated attacks of pneumonia, failed to respond to several injections of a standard pneumococcal polysaccharide vaccine. What was wrong with him and what did his physician do?

Here are some suggestions for your answer:

1. Pauling was the most famous proponent of the *instructive* or *template* theory, while Burnet thought out the *clonal selection* theory, to which everyone now subscribes. The problems for instructive theories were (1) different antibodies do not in fact have the same amino acid sequence, (2) they could not ex-

plain memory or tolerance, (3) once the genetic code was understood there was no mechanism for an antigen to induce a permanent change in DNA, (4) eventually it was shown that individual lymphocytes recognized different antigens. The problem for clonal selection was considered to be that it was incredibly wasteful to carry around millions of lymphocytes that might never be used. However, this was a short-sighted argument because the world of microorganisms is constantly throwing up new antigenic types and selecting the most successful; Burnet's theory simply says that the immune system does the same. As he himself said: 'It is a Darwinian approach.'

2. For clonal selection to work, each lymphocyte (B or T) must retain its specific antigen receptor through numerous divisions, otherwise some members of the clone would be no use against the original triggering antigen. Thus in each B cell, only one combination of V, D, and J genes is chosen to code for the immunoglubulin heavy chain (and only one for the light chain). However, it cannot be known in advance which class of Ig (i.e. which type of Fc region) will be most effective; IgM, IgG, IgA, and IgE all have their advantages in particular situations. Therefore every B cell must retain the ability to switch classes—from IgM to IgG, etc.—without losing its antigen specificity.

3. Purely from the viewpoint of the immune system, this statement appears to be true. The function of MHC molecules is to display antigenic peptides on the surface of cells in such a way that T cells recognize them and take appropriate action—cytotoxicity in the case of class I MHC and help in the case of class II. In the thymus, MHC molecules play a major part in deciding which T cell receptors are to be deleted and which 'permitted'. If T cells had not evolved, there would seem to be no point in displaying MHC in the thymus or MHC–peptide complexes on B cells, macrophages, etc. However, it has been suggested that MHC molecules have other, non-immunological roles, for example in cell association in primitive animals and even in mating preference (dogs can unerringly smell and distinguish foreign MHC molecules in urine).

4. Clearly antigenic variation contributes to the success of many pathogens in avoiding elimination by the immune system, including some that might otherwise have great difficulty surviving, such as the African trypanosome living free in the blood. It is also presumably useful to organisms that may need to infect the same host repeatedly, such as influenza in man. But there is no reason to suppose that *all* successful pathogens need to vary their antigens—though those that do not may run the risk of being eliminated by vaccination campaigns, as smallpox was. (It might be worth pointing out that the attenuated viruses used as vaccines are selected for variation of virulence but *not* of surface antigens.) Another point of interest is that not all antigenic variation is driven by the immune system; the free-living protozoan *Paramecium* varies its surface antigens in response to temperature, salinity, etc. without ever having to worry about immunity.

5. Certainly memory is one of the unique and valuable features of the lymphocyte, but not the most characteristic. Some extremely useful lymphocyte functions, such as the IgM response to bacterial polysaccharides, do not show memory at all. Recirculation is probably equally important, since without it antigen and lymphocyte would seldom meet. But the real hallmark of the lymphocyte is *specificity*, which can in turn be traced back to rearrangement of receptor genes. Whether the immunoglobulin or T cell receptor genes are in the coding (rearranged) or germ-line (non-rearranged), configuration is the clinching test of whether the cell in question is a B cell, a T cell, or neither.

6. There is much truth in this, though often the damage is trivial and rapidly repaired—the one-day runny nose in some colds for example. However, by definition a pathogen implies *disease*, and disease implies tissue damage. The important thing is that many of the symptoms of disease *are* side-effects of the processes that lead to elimination of the pathogen (or sometimes fail to achieve this). Only in the case of microbial toxins or direct cell destruction can one say that the symptoms are nothing to do with the immune system.

7. This is the celebrated case in which Bruton (1953) first demonstrated the association between repeated bacterial infection and absence of gammaglobulins in an electrophoretic analysis of serum. The boy lacked B cells, a condition now known as Bruton's agammaglobulinaemia which, because it is caused by a gene on the X chromosome, is inherited by boys from their mothers. Chickenpox, a viral disease, was no problem because his T cells were normal. Monthly injections of pooled normal human gammaglobulin kept him healthy—the treatment still used today.

Part 3

The host–pathogen balance

26 Epidemiology

In the previous sections of this book, we described the world of pathogens and that of the immune system, treating each element more or less in isolation. However, the real world does not consist of clean cages of highly inbred mice exposed under laboratory conditions to a single clone of identical pathogens, but of large groups of individuals, genetically different and living in different circumstances, irregularly exposed to a large array of pathogens, also genetically highly variable and frequently interacting among themselves. In this last section we consider this balance between human populations and their pathogens with two crucial aims in mind: (1) to *understand* the 'real world' situation, and (2) where necessary to try and *control* it. In the three following chapters we discuss the available control strategies; here we shall look at some of the factors that determine the incidence and distribution of infectious diseases—that is, their *epidemiology*.

The science of epidemiology has developed a language of its own, and Table 26.1 lists some of the terms commonly used by workers in this field.

Diagnosing, monitoring, and predicting disease

In order to study the epidemiology of an infectious disease, one must first be confident of being able to diagnose it. Diagnosis can be clinical, microbiological, or immunological.

1. *Clinical diagnosis* is often easy, particularly during epidemics (e.g. childhood virus infections), in endemic areas (e.g. malaria during the transmission season), or when the symptoms and signs are characteristic (e.g. elephantiasis). However, clinical diagnosis is an art rather than a science; it is never absolutely precise and—especially in children—frequently wrong.

2. *Microbiological* diagnosis is usually precise, but it must be remembered that finding a pathogen does not prove it is causing the disease in question. The methods used include simple microscopy with or without special stains (for bacteria, fungi, protozoa), culture in agar media (mainly for bacteria, particularly for assessing antibiotic sensitivity) or in animal cells (for viruses), electron microscopy (for viruses), and DNA/RNA sequencing (mainly for studying variation). The use of monoclonal antibodies, usually coupled to

Table 26.1 The language of epidemiology

Prevalence	The proportion (%) of individuals with an attribute (e.g. disease, antibody) in a population
Incidence	The number of new events (e.g. disease, seroconversion) in a susceptible population
Seroprevalence	The proportion of antibody- or antigen-positive individuals
Seroconversion	The detection of antibody or antigen for the first time
Endemic	Constantly present in the population
Epidemic	Occurring in an unusually high incidence in a population
Pandemic	A worldwide epidemic
Sporadic	Apparently unrelated cases (i.e. not epidemic)
Outbreak	One or more new cases in a single area, possibly related
Incubation period	Time between exposure and symptoms
Reproduction rate	Average number of susceptible individuals infected by a single case (often referred to as R_0)
Subclinical infection	Disease with few or no symptoms
Carrier	An infected individual, who may be symptomless, able to infect others
Reservoir	A site from which infection may originate
Zoonosis	An infection with an animal reservoir
Vector	A living agent transmitting a pathogen
Nosocomial	Acquired in hospital
Mortality	The prevalence or incidence of death in a population
Morbidity	The prevalence of disease in a population
Herd immunity	Resistance in a population due to some, but not all, being immune
Quarantine	Restriction of movement to prevent spread
Retrospective study	Comparison of groups, measured retrospectively
Prospective study	Planned comparison of groups following exposure

fluorescent dyes, allows extremely rapid and specific identification of pathogens and their antigens. Detection of antigen is particularly helpful as it denotes an ongoing infection.

3. *Immunological* diagnosis is valuable when the pathogen is hard to find or to identify. It is essentially retrospective and does not prove the presence of an infection, merely that it has occurred. The principal responses measured are specific antibody, T cell proliferation/cytokine release, and skin tests. Since B and T cells recognize *antigens* rather than whole pathogens, there is sometimes the problem of cross-reaction, but immunological screening can be very

useful in monitoring the spread of epidemics and the success of vaccine campaigns. In addition, antibodies are most useful for detecting microbial antigens in the laboratory (see above).

Theoretical epidemiology

In the age of the computer, it has become possible to create mathematical models of disease spread, given certain basic numerical values. These include: the number of susceptible individuals in a population, the duration of the infectious state, the distance over which spread occurs, and in the case of vector-borne diseases, the duration of the infectious state for the vector. Models of this kind have been particularly valuable in predicting the periodicity of epidemics and the proportion of a population that would need to be immunized, or of animals that would need to be culled (see prion disease, Chapters 7 and 30) in order for a disease to die out, and in general their calculations have agreed closely with already known facts. For example the elimination of measles would require a vaccination uptake of at least 95% whereas smallpox was eradicated with only about 80% of the world's population being vaccinated. Mathematical models are also useful in planning drug trials where drug resistance is expected.

Practical epidemiology

The epidemiology of any given disease depends on four main factors:

(1) the *host* and its variables—lifestyle, immune competence, genetics;

(2) the *pathogen* and its variables—virulence factors, genetics;

(3) the degree of *contact* between the two, which depends on the numbers of pathogens in the environment and the means by which they spread.

(4) the effect, if any, of *treatment* or *preventive measures* (vaccines, drugs, public health strategy). We shall illustrate these points in relation to three diseases, one viral (AIDS), one bacterial (TB), and one protozoal (malaria), which together make up a large percentage of the total world burden of morbidity and mortality caused by infection, and all of which are at present on the increase.

HIV and AIDS (2.6 million deaths per year)

It is estimated that following a single exposure to HIV, there is up to a 10% chance of becoming infected—a much lower rate than that of the common childhood viruses, which is almost 100%. The rate of disease progression is then related to the total viral load, and is monitored mainly by following T cell numbers in the blood. As far as can be judged (the virus was only identified 20 years ago and the first contact between this animal virus and human populations probably occurred not more than about 50 years ago) the morbidity and mortality in those infected and not treated are very close to 100%, the exceptions being mainly individuals genetically lacking the 'second receptor' for the virus. One can imagine that if humans were exposed to HIV for long enough, this defective genotype, having a strong survival advantage, would spread quite rapidly through the populations at risk, as the sickle gene appears to have (see malaria, below). At present the very high morbidity and mortality are due to two main causes: the severe damage to the immune system, which limits effective immunity, both against HIV itself and against a whole range of *opportunists*, and the extremely high level of antigenic variation, which renders what immunity there is against HIV ineffective and vaccination difficult. Only two strategies of control are currently available: limitation of *contact* and *chemotherapy* (see Table 25.5). Monitoring is by peripheral T cell counts and the detection of complications (see Table 25.6).

AIDS is one of the few diseases to have emerged within living memory (see Chapter 35 for a discussion of some others) and the observations that unravelled its pathogenesis are a good example of epidemiology in action. The alarm was given by a sharp rise in the incidence of pneumonia due to *Pneumocystis carinii*, previously considered a harmless parasite (1981). Other opportunistic infections were noted in the same individuals, along with skin tumours (Kaposi's sarcoma), low blood T cell counts, and severe weight loss. Evidently a new form of immunodeficiency had suddenly appeared. Consideration of the type of patient affected revealed that they were mostly either (a) male homosexuals, (b) intravenous drug abusers, or (c) haemophiliacs requiring injections of human clotting factor VIII. Clearly the common element was the transfer of blood or body fluids, which immediately suggested an infectious agent, and by 1983 a French group had identified a virus, later baptized HIV (now HIV-1). Since this time the balance of infection has shifted so that heterosexual transmission is now the most common route. Sequencing of the HIV genome and comparison with other viruses strongly suggested an origin in African primates. It is a frustrating thought that, with the possible exception of mother–child transfer, all the means by which HIV spreads could *theoretically* be prevented by changes in human behaviour, such as promoting safe sex and the avoidance of needle sharing. By contrast, infections transmitted by the aerosol route (e.g. tuberculosis) are almost impossible to avoid.

Tuberculosis (1.5 million deaths per year)

Here the picture is quite different. Unlike AIDS, TB is an ancient scourge of mankind. *M. tuberculosis* is fairly common in the air we breathe, and it is estimated that one-third of the world population is infected. However, less than

10% of these individuals show symptoms, while in many others the development of a positive skin (Mantoux) test indicates that they have responded immunologically and acquired a level of cell-mediated immunity to the bacteria—without having eliminated them completely, because a change of general health status can be sufficient to 'light up' the disease (see below). Disease activity is monitored clinically, radiologically, and microbiologically, a positive sputum being a particular danger sign because of the risk of infecting others. This precarious balance between host and pathogen is mainly due to the ability of the bacteria to survive inside phagocytic cells and even inside granulomas composed of large numbers of phagocytes and other immunological cells; antigenic variation between pathogen strains does not seem to be a major factor.

On the other hand many variables influence the ability of the host to keep the infection down, of which the most important appear to be: (1) the general level of immune competence, which can be compromised by malnutrition, stress, other diseases, and particularly HIV infection (see Chapter 25 for a discussion of this and other secondary immunodeficiencies); (2) the widely used BCG vaccine, which undoubtedly gives some protection at the population level, though more effectively in children and to a very different extent in different countries; (3) the presence of other mycobacteria in the local environment, which may affect the response to both TB itself and to the BCG vaccine; (4) genetic differences between individuals, affecting mainly intracellular pathogens. These include mutations in the IFNγ receptor and IL-12 genes, the transporter gene Slc11a1 (see Chapter 8) and, more weakly, the HLA class II allele DR2 and numerous other candidate genes.

Before the days of antibiotics, treatment of active TB relied on the isolating and restful effect of sanatoria, usually at high altitude, but the present level of control has been largely achieved by BCG, together with chemotherapy, which both kills the organisms and reduces transmission. Streptomycin, PAS, isoniazid, rifampicin, and ethambutol have been used, generally long-term and in triple combinations. None of these drugs are infallible and all have side-effects, and with the spread of HIV around the tropics and the emergence of antibiotic-resistant strains, TB threatens to be once again a major killer, as it was a century ago. Indeed the co-existence of HIV and *M. tuberculosis* in a population represents pathogen–pathogen interaction at its worst.

Malaria (1.1 million deaths per year)

Caused by four species of the protozoon *Plasmodium*, this disease is normally restricted to tropical areas by the distribution of the *Anopheles* mosquito vector, which plays an essential role in the pathogen's complex life-cycle. However, the huge increase in migration and travel (2 000 000 people are estimated to cross a national boundary every day) means that cases of malaria are increasingly seen in the non-tropical world, and non-travellers have occasionally been infected by mosquitoes that have made the journey from an endemic area by aeroplane. The only reliable diagnostic marker is the finding of parasites in a blood film.

In the endemic areas themselves, the pattern of disease is determined by numerous factors:

(1) The distribution of the *vector*—at low altitudes and near swampy water.

(2) The *age* of the infected individual; young children harbour more parasites and are more likely to die of complications such as anaemia and cerebral malaria, probably because of the slow development of immunity. Adults that have acquired a partial level of immunity sufficient to keep parasite numbers low and symptoms absent can lose this after 6 months abroad, suggesting that repeated boosting is required to maintain protection.

(3) Extensive surface antigenic variation by the blood-stage parasite, to the point where every member of a village may carry a different variant; this variability is enhanced by the possession of a clear sexual stage in the parasite life-cycle, allowing rapid reassortment of parasite genes.

(4) Genetic differences between individuals. The latter may operate at the level of the red cell: absence of the Duffy blood group antigen prevents the entry of *P. vivax*, while heterozygotes for HbS (the sickle-cell trait) show partial resistance to *P. falciparum*. The latter has had the interesting effect of helping to maintain what is otherwise a deleterious gene in endemic areas, at the expense of those unfortunate enough to be homozygous, who suffer life-threatening sickle-cell anaemia—a good example of *balanced polymorphism*. There is also a link between severity and HLA type, probably mainly due to linkage between alleles of the HLA and TNF genes; TNF is thought to play a role in both protection and disease.

Malaria displays important interactions with other infections. It is immunosuppressive (though much less so than HIV) and even mild malaria has been shown to interfere with the effectiveness of vaccines against *S. pneumoniae* and *N. meningitidis*. It also appears to be a co-factor, along with EB virus, for the development of Burkitt's lymphoma. Here the mechanism is not so clear, but suppression of the CTL response to virus-infected B cells may be one element. Since the realization that vector control (e.g. by DDT) is not as simple as was thought, numerous other strategies have been tried. Experimental vaccines have been devised against the liver stage, the infected red cell, the free (merozoite) blood parasite, and even the sexual stage (to block transmission by preventing the mosquito stage). However, effective control still relies on minimizing contact (by mosquito nets, etc.) and the careful use of chemotherapy; unfortunately drug resistance has occurred to virtually every drug and the pharmaceutical industry is engaged in a literal race against the pathogen.

The value of epidemiology

We have looked at only three diseases and there are dozens of others, each with its special and interesting epidemiological features (see Chapters 30–34). What is the use of all this knowledge? The answer is that without it, the chances of controlling any infectious disease would be practically nil. A classic example is the detective work carried out in 1855 by the London doctor John Snow, who used detailed maps of disease incidence and the London water supplies to pinpoint the source of cholera, hitherto rampant in some parts of the city. This was a case where *public health* measures were clearly called for. On the other hand the massive incidence of soil-derived tetanus during the early months of trench warfare in the First World War—a disease already known to be due to a toxin that could be neutralised by antibody—was an indication for passive immunization with antibody, soon to be replaced by active immunization by a *vaccine*. Finally, the susceptibility of the ever-present staphylococcus to penicillin and the non-availability of a vaccine was the impetus for the modern science of *chemotherapy*. In the next three chapters we shall look at these three contrasting ways of controlling infectious disease.

27 Control of infectious disease: vaccination

Immunization makes use of the ability of the adaptive immune system to learn and improve. It may be *active*, inducing the immune system itself to acquire a permanently enhanced resistance to a particular pathogen, or *passive*, where preformed immune components (usually antibody) are introduced into the patient (see later). Active immunization directed at a specific organism is known as *vaccination*, in commemoration of Edward Jenner's pioneering work (1797) on the prevention of smallpox by scarification with vaccinia (cowpox). Smallpox has now been eradicated (1980) but ever since Pasteur showed in the 1880s that it was possible to immunize against other infections, the general term 'vaccination' has been retained.

The function of a vaccine is to induce *memory* without causing *disease*, so that the pathogen itself, on first contact with the patient, provokes a secondary rather than a primary response, and a response of the right kind to be effective, i.e. antibody or T cell-mediated, systemic or mucosal. In general, vaccines are more successful when mimicking a normally effective immune response (e.g. measles) than when trying to improve partial or absent immunity (e.g. TB, HIV). The aim of a vaccine is ideally to prevent *infection* occurring at all, but there are special situations, e.g. vector-borne diseases like malaria and leishmaniasis, where a vaccine that only prevents *transmission* has been contemplated.

Requirements for a vaccine

There are not vaccines for every disease; this is because a vaccine, to be worth bringing into use, must satisfy four criteria. It must be (1) effective, (2) safe, (3) stable, (4) affordable.

Effectiveness

The best vaccines are very effective indeed. As mentioned above, Jenner's cowpox vaccine eventually eliminated smallpox, and several other viral diseases have been targeted by World Health Organization for eradication within the next generation; these include measles, rubella, mumps, and polio. Whether or not this is achieved, there is no doubt that in the developed world these four diseases are rapidly disappearing, and the same is true for the 'toxic' bacterial diseases tetanus and diphtheria (Fig. 27.1). It is estimated that vaccination currently saves some 3 million lives per year—a figure that could increase to 5 million if vaccines were universally available.

At the other end of the scale, there are vaccines that, though undoubtedly beneficial, stand no chance at present of eradicating the corresponding disease;

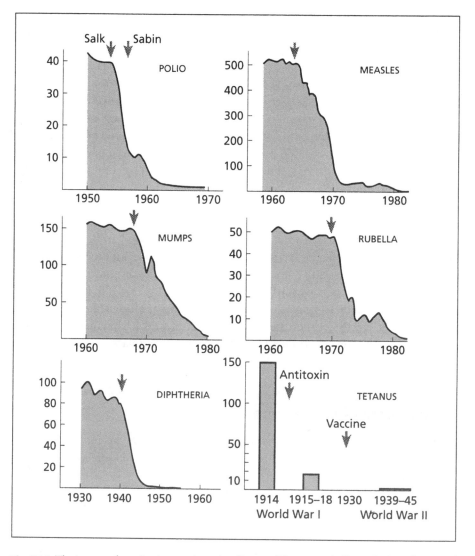

Fig. 27.1 The impact of vaccination on six major diseases. The arrows indicate the introduction of general immunization in each case. Polio, measles, mumps, rubella, cases per 10 000 in the USA; diphtheria, cases per million in the UK; tetanus, cases per 10 000 in British Army troops (also showing the dramatic protective effect of passive antibody).

examples are influenza, rabies, and BCG (the TB vaccine). Note that it may not always be necessary to vaccinate every single member of the population for two reasons: (1) when most individuals are protected and few are susceptible, transmission becomes increasingly difficult and may eventually die out ('*herd immunity*'); (2) an attenuated strain may actually replace the pathogenic type in the environment, as is happening with polio in water supplies, so that individuals become immunized without knowing it.

The reasons for reduced effectiveness differ. In the case of influenza, antigenic variation (see Fig. 21.2) makes it hard to match the vaccine to the current virus strain. With rabies, there is a vast animal reservoir beyond the reach of the vaccinator. With BCG, the problem is that it works much better in some parts of the world than others, for reasons that are not fully understood but probably reflect the influence of other mycobacteria in the local environment as well as genetic differences between human populations. However, the use of BCG is so universal that it would be ethically and politically difficult to replace it experimentally with an alternative.

Individual genetic differences, particularly in HLA antigens with their role in presenting peptides to T cells (see Chapter 17), can determine the success or failure of vaccines based on small peptides, making a 'universal' vaccine—for example to malaria—rather unlikely. In most cases a 'cocktail' or a conjugate of different peptides will be necessary. Polysaccharide vaccines are inefficient at inducing memory, but this can be overcome by coupling them to a protein carrier—either one from the same organism (e.g. *H. influenzae*) or one to which most people would be primed (e.g. tetanus toxoid). Finally, there are diseases where no vaccine is currently available at all: leading examples are the common cold, staphylococcal infections, and virtually all fungal, protozoal, and worm infections. The reason is usually technical, but may also be economic. Opportunist infections, against which healthy individuals do not need to be vaccinated (e.g. CMV, pneumocystis) are a special case; it will be interesting to see whether vaccination in the early stages of immunodeficiency will delay the onset of the opportunistic infection. Table 27.1 summarizes the major diseases for which effective vaccines currently do and do not exist.

Safety

This is an increasingly critical consideration. One must remember that vaccines are the only medical treatment administered to perfectly healthy people, and 'vaccine accidents'—real or imaginary—can lead to public alarm and enormously expensive litigation. Live attenuated vaccines are the most vulnerable because of the real possibility of reversion to the pathogenic 'wild' type. Here established vaccines differ enormously: BCG is estimated to have lost 100 genes from the wild-type *M. bovis*, whereas some polio vaccine strains have mutations in ten or less (see below). Other important safety problems are listed in Table 27.2.

Table 27.1 The main vaccines in use, with some important diseases where vaccines are still lacking. Vaccines bracketed together are usually given simultaneously

	Virus	Bacteria	Fungi	Protozoa or worms
In general use	Polio Measles Mumps Rubella Hepatitis B	Diphtheria Tetanus Pertussis BCG (in tropics)		
Mainly for those 'at risk'	Influenza Yellow fever Hepatitis A Rabies Varicella– zoster Rotavirus	BCG Cholera Typhoid *Pneumococcus* *Meningococcus* *Haemophilus* Plague Anthrax		

Vaccines not available	Adenovirus
	Rhinovirus
	Herpesviruses
	Respiratory
	  syncytial virus
	*HIV
		Staphylococcus
		Gp A *Streptococcus*
		Gonococcus
		Syphilis
		**Leprosy
		Chlamydia
			Candida
			Pneumocystis
			Cryptococcus,
			  etc.
				*Malaria
				Leishmania
				Trypanosomiasis
				Schistosomiasis
				Filariasis

* Trials have been carried out with experimental vaccines.
** BCG gives some protection against leprosy.

Table 27.2 The main safety problems with vaccines. Those asterisked are the most important. In general, living attenuated vaccines are not given to immunodeficient patients

The vaccine
   *Attenuated organisms revert to wild type (e.g. polio types 2, 3)
   'Killed' organisms not properly killed (has happened with polio)
   Inclusion of toxic material (e.g. typhoid, pertussis)
   Contamination by animal viruses
   Contamination by egg proteins (hypersensitivity)
   Cross-reaction with 'self' (autoimmunity)

The patient
   *Immunodeficiency (attenuated organisms may cause serious/fatal disease)
   Local inflammatory reactions, often to the adjuvant
   Worsening of disease by increasing immunopathology
   Hypersensitivity to vaccine (e.g. tetanus)
   Interference between vaccines given together (not always)
   Induction of inappropriate response (e.g. respiratory syncytial virus, dengue)
   Patient already exposed (therapeutic vaccination, e.g. HIV)

Partly for these reasons, and partly because of the low profitability of vaccines compared to chemotherapy (see Chapter 28), many pharmaceutical companies nowadays are cautious of embarking on vaccine development.

Stability

This becomes particularly important where vaccines are used far from their site of manufacture, and is again chiefly a problem of living vaccines (see below).

Affordability

Most vaccines are remarkably cheap; indeed, vaccination has been called the most cost-effective form of preventive medicine ever invented. For example, the cost of vaccinating a child against measles, pertussis, diphtheria, tetanus, polio, and tuberculosis is less than $20. However, it must be borne in mind that for some tropical countries, even a few pence per person per year may exceed the available health budget. Moreover, some vaccines are definitely not cheap; the hepatitis B vaccine still costs around $60 per individual—having fallen from $125! To introduce a *new* vaccine is extremely expensive (see later).

Established vaccines

To induce memory requires exposure of the immune system to an antigen or set of antigens identical or closely similar to those on the infectious organism. This can be achieved in a number of ways, some established and some still experimental (Table 27.3). For practical purposes, the essential distinction is between *living* and *non-living* vaccines.

Living vaccines have been outstandingly successful with viral diseases, from smallpox onwards. In fact, smallpox was unusual in that an animal virus existed with sufficient antigenic similarity to immunize (mainly via T cells) against the human disease, but which was unable to survive more than a few weeks in the human host. The same principle has been tried with some other viruses (e.g. rotavirus), but without comparable success; a similar concept underlies the once-favoured use of the vole bacillus to immunize against human TB, and of the practice of leishmanization, in which a deliberately induced cutaneous infection gave some protection against the more serious visceral leishmaniasis.

The alternative approach is to *attenuate* a normal human pathogen, which was originally a process of inducing random mutation by imposing unusual growth conditions (low temperature, abnormal host cell, etc.) and selecting out the mutants that have lost virulence but retained antigenicity. A better way to do this nowadays is through recombinant DNA technology and sequencing of the full genome, allowing the deliberate deletion of, for example, known virulence

Table 27.3 The antigens used in vaccination are of various kinds. Some examples are given of each type

Type of antigen	Examples
(1) Whole organisms	
living (e.g. from animals)	Vaccinia (for smallpox)
killed	Rabies, influenza, polio (Salk), hepatitis A, pertussis, Typhoid, cholera
(2) Attenuated (i.e. mutant) organisms	
randomly	Measles, mumps, rubella, polio (Sabin), yellow fever, varicella–zoster, BCG, typhoid
*site-directed	Cholera, typhoid
(3) Antigenic fragments	
inactivated toxins (toxoids)	Tetanus, diphtheria
capsular polysaccharides	Meningococcus, pneumococcus Haemophilus influenza
Surface antigen	Hepatitis B
bacterial pili	*Gonococcus, *E. coli
(4) Peptides	
gene-cloned	Hepatitis B, *malaria
synthetic	Foot-and-mouth disease (cattle)
(5) *Genes cloned into living vectors	*HIV in vaccinia
(6) *DNA	*Influenza, *malaria, *TB
(7) *Anti-idiotype antibodies	*Bacterial LPS

* Still experimental, i.e. used in trials or animal models only.

factors or undesired antigens as well as reducing the risk of reversion. However, the existing attenuated viral vaccines were all produced by the original approach (aptly termed 'genetic roulette'). Only one bacterial vaccine has been produced by attenuation—the *bacille Calmette-Guérin* (BCG) for TB, which took over 10 years and 200 passages of *M. bovis* to develop.

Living vaccines are in general more immunogenic because they are still capable of some growth and they tend to locate to the site where protection is required; for example the oral (Sabin) polio vaccine induces better intestinal IgA levels than the killed (Salk) vaccine, which is injected intramuscularly. However, live vaccines suffer from three drawbacks: instability if a complete '*cold chain*' is not maintained from factory to clinic; the danger of *reversion* to the non-mutant (wild) type and their ability to cause serious disease in *immunodeficient* individuals (Table 27.2). In the days of smallpox vaccination, the first sign of severe T-cell deficiency (see Fig. 24.1) was sometimes the development of spreading and eventually fatal infections with the supposedly non-virulent vaccinia virus, and these babies, if given BCG, risk dying of 'disseminated' BCG-osis'—effectively a new, man-made disease. A reminder of the danger was the death from vaccinia of three patients in Zaire, immunized with the virus containing a cloned antigen from HIV as part of an attempt to protect against AIDS. Reversion was seen in some early polio vaccine campaigns, which was subsequently explained by the discovery that some of the original 'attenuated' strains (Types 2 and 3) contained only two new mutations; in contrast, Type 1 contained 57 mutations and has not reverted. On the other hand, *over*-attenuation would be self-defeating, since the vaccine might not behave like the live infection in which case it would, in effect, be 'dead'.

In contrast, non-living vaccines are relatively safe. They range from whole organisms killed by heat, formalin, β–propiolactone, etc. to small portions of an organism carrying the critical antigens; for example the polysaccharide capsules of *Streptococcus pneumoniae*, the surface coat of the hepatitis B virus, or the inactivated toxins ('toxoids') of the tetanus and diphtheria bacilli (Table 27.3). Since the injected antigen does not proliferate or localize in the way a living vaccine can, killed vaccines are generally less immunogenic and need to be given more than once, usually by intramuscular injection and often with an *adjuvant* (see below). The safety problems are restricted to (1) failure to kill the organisms properly, and (2) the inclusion of toxic material; the well-known (but never absolutely proved) risks with the whooping-cough vaccine may be associated with the *Bordetella pertussis* endotoxin (Fig. 27.2). There is the further problem that a more purified antigen, lacking the 'pathogen-associated

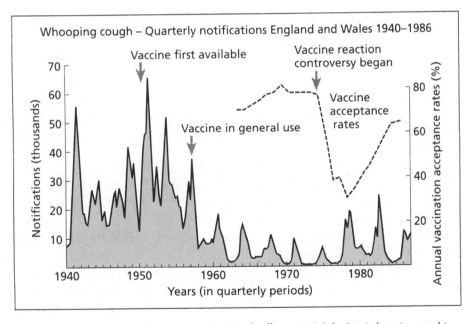

Fig. 27.2 The introduction of a vaccine against *Bordetella pertussis* infection (whooping cough), which reached about 90 per cent of the population by 1956, reduced the incidence of the disease dramatically, though periodic epidemics still occurred. Anxiety that the vaccine could cause serious neurological reactions led to a fall in the numbers vaccinated and a prompt increase in cases (1978, 1982), some fatal. This illustrates both the medical and the social aspect of vaccination. (With acknowledgement to Dr N. S. Galbraith and the PHLS Communicable Disease Surveillance Centre, London.)

molecular patterns' of the whole organism (see Chapter 11), may not trigger an optimal response through failure to activate innate immunity.

Experimental vaccine strategies

Vaccine development is currently at a very interesting stage thanks to several promising new molecular biological techniques (see Table 27.3). First in the field was the production of protein antigens by *recombinant DNA* methods; the present hepatitis B vaccine, made by cloning the gene for the surface antigen in yeast, has replaced the original vaccine derived from the blood of carriers of the disease. Alternatively, small *peptides* can be produced synthetically, as has been shown in animals with a foot-and-mouth disease capsid protein—though here, as mentioned above, host genotypic variation may become an important factor. An advantage of this method is that epitopes aimed at B and T cells can be coupled together in appropriate proportions—for example four of each.

An alternative approach is to insert the desired gene into a living virus or bacterium (suitably attenuated) which, administered as a vaccine, will express and induce immunity to the inserted protein. Vaccinia and many other viruses, and also some bacteria (salmonella, BCG), have been proposed as '*vaccine vectors*'. The latest development along this line is to inject the gene itself—the '*DNA vaccine*'—coupled to a suitable promoter, intramuscularly; surprisingly, muscle cells will express the corresponding protein and induce immunity. DNA vaccines on their own have been somewhat disappointing, but DNA vaccination followed by a protein or live vector—the 'prime-boost' strategy—may be a good way to induce cytotoxic (CD8) T cell immunity, which might be important in the case of HIV, TB, etc. The recent surge of interest in genomics (see Chapter 8) has greatly facilitated the search for genes and/or proteins with selected suitable qualities for vaccine candidates.

Another novel approach, for use with vector-borne diseases, is the 'transmission-blocking vaccine' (see Fig. 27.3). Finally, one should mention the possibility of using antibodies as antigens—the '*anti-idiotype*' strategy, which depends on the fact that antibodies made against other antibodies can sometimes actually mimic the three-dimensional shape of the original antigen. This approach seems to many far-fetched, but might be of use with antigens that are not themselves very immunogenic, for example the lipid A portion of endotoxin (see Figs 3.2, 31.1) and perhaps other lipid and polysaccharide-based molecules which, though immunogenic, do not normally induce memory and the switch to IgG typical of proteins (see Chapter 18).

Long- and short-term vaccines

One exception to the rule that a vaccine must induce memory occurs when the requirement for protection is only temporary (the 'tourist vaccine'). For example

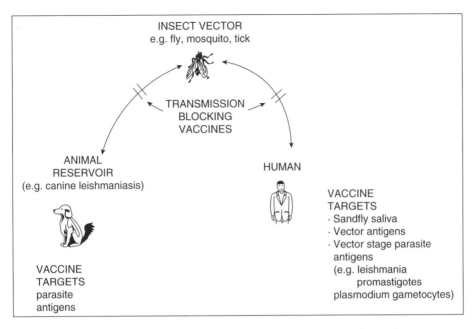

INSECT VECTOR
e.g. fly, mosquito, tick

TRANSMISSION
BLOCKING
VACCINES

ANIMAL
RESERVOIR
(e.g. canine leishmaniasis)

HUMAN

VACCINE
TARGETS
· Sandfly saliva
· Vector antigens
· Vector stage parasite
  antigens
  (e.g. leishmania
        promastigotes
  plasmodium gametocytes)

VACCINE
TARGETS
parasite
antigens

Fig. 27.3 Strategies for transmission-blocking vaccination for vector-borne diseases.

the induction of a strong primary antibody response, even without any memory, would be enough to protect against many infections for 3–6 months, though another course would be needed for a subsequent visit. This is probably how most polysaccharide vaccines work. In fact the apparent life-long duration of protection by some infections (e.g. mumps, measles) may be slightly misleading, since recovered individuals will be regularly 'boosted' by exposure to infected contacts; the same process would also make the duration of protection by a vaccine appear more permanent than it really was. Here the danger is that as the disease is progressively eliminated from the population, as measles, etc. may soon be, this boosting will disappear and vaccination may need to be repeated more often. Boosting is already recommended for vaccines where there is no regular exposure, e.g. every 10 years for tetanus.

Route of vaccination

Until recently, vaccines were given intramuscularly, with the exception of the attenuated polio vaccine which is given orally. In fact the oral route should be ideal for all pathogens that enter via the intestine (as polio does), so that immunity is generated where it is most needed. Intranasal and inhaled vaccines have also been tried experimentally for appropriate pathogens. It is even possible to express viral antigens in plants, which might lead to the attractive prospect of an edible vaccine.

When and whom to vaccinate

In general, vaccines are given as early as possible, with certain qualifications. BCG, given at birth in tropical countries, is delayed until school entry where the risk of exposure to TB is less. The measles, mumps, rubella vaccine is delayed for at least a year to allow maternally transmitted antibody to disappear, because this would otherwise reduce vaccine efficiency. Some vaccines are restricted to those 'at risk'—for example, *Streptococcus pneumoniae* for the elderly, influenza when an epidemic is expected, yellow fever for travellers to endemic areas, etc.

Adjuvants

Often an immune response and/or the development of memory can be enhanced if another substance is injected together with the antigen. It was discovered 70 years ago that aluminium salts had this property, and vaccines such as the tetanus and diphtheria toxoids are still given in an emulsion with aluminium hydroxide as an *adjuvant*. Probably their main effect is to induce local inflammation and retain the antigen for a longer period, but excessive inflammation, as was seen in animals given Complete Freund's Adjuvant, would not be clinically acceptable. However, other mechanisms are possible, and new-generation adjuvants are being developed, based on improved understanding of antigen presentation and the role of dendritic cells and cytokines. Indeed, some cytokines themselves have considerable adjuvant activity (IL-1, IL-2, IL-12, IFNγ). The artificial lipid vesicles known as *liposomes*, used for drug delivery and also in the cosmetic industry, and the somewhat similar immunostimulating complexes (ISCOMs), have had some success as vehicles to transport antigens into antigen-presenting cells. Some enterotoxins (*E. coli*, cholera) have shown promise as adjuvants for mucosal vaccines while plasmid DNA has its own adjuvanticity.

Development and testing

Development of a new vaccine proceeds along fairly standard lines. Candidate preparations are first tested in suitable small animals if available (generally mice or rabbits), often followed by a trial in a non-human primate, looking for a significant degree of protection, a lack of side-effects, and if possible a correlation between protection and some 'marker'—that is, a laboratory test such as antibody levels or cytokine production that can be used to follow responses in human populations (since it will not usually be ethical to deliberately infect them). Finally, a series of clinical trials will be carried out, of increasing size and stringency, as shown in Table 27.4. Whether a vaccine will be considered

Table 27.4 Stages in the testing of a candidate vaccine

Animal	Aim	Comments
Mouse	Experimental model	Defined genetics and immune response; mutant strains available, but diseases may not always resemble the human equivalent
Rabbit guinea-pig hamster, etc.	Intermediate model	May be better mimic of human pathology (e.g. guinea-pig tuberculosis), but immunity less well characterized than for mouse
Non-human primates	Human surrogate	Closest to human for immunity, toxicity, but expensive and difficult to handle; also not genetically defined
Human		
Phase I	Safety; side-effects dose range	Small numbers of patients (e.g. 10)
Phase II	Safety, efficacy	Intermediate numbers (10–100); randomized, placebo-controlled double-blind trial where possible
Phase III	Large-scale; comparison with standard therapy	Multi-centre (100–1000 patients)
Phase IV	Long-term efficacy, cost, safety in specific patient groups	Analysis of multiple trials following general public release

successful will ultimately depend on the balance between reduction in mortality and/or morbidity on the one hand and cost, safety, and the global importance of the disease on the other. A cheap but only partially protective vaccine against malaria or HIV would probably be pursued, while an expensive and wholly protective one against Lassa fever might not. It is estimated that the cost of developing, testing, and delivering a new vaccine today would be in the region of $300 million.

Passive ('immediate') immunization

As most people who have lived in the tropics know, the acute treatment for snakebite is to inject antivenom, which is simply *antibody* made in advance against the relevant toxin in a horse or goat. The same principle is used for some acute infections, particularly those due to exotoxin-secreting bacteria. There are also a few other indications, the most interesting being rabies, where a combination of passive antibody and active immunization is used, the antibody to mop up virus before it gets into the nerves, the vaccine to induce a host antibody response during the slow passage to the brain, which can take about 6 weeks. The 'last-minute' tourist injection of anti-hepatitis A antibody and the monthly injections of pooled normal human immunoglobulin for agammaglobulinaemia (see Chapter 24) also come into this category. Passive immunization is usually carried out using *polyclonal* antisera from either immunized animals or convalescent humans, which have the advantage of multiple specificity and isotype but the disadvantage of low activity and short supply. *Monoclonal* antibodies (mAbs) could be available in unlimited amounts but their specificity for a single antigenic determinant means that in practice mixtures of several mAbs would be needed. At present the only mAb in clinical use is against respiratory syncytial virus.

The frightening recent development of bio-terrorism may prove to be the most valuable application of passive immunotherapy, and it has been suggested that pools of mAbs against the toxins of anthrax, botulism, etc., and viruses such as smallpox and Ebola, should be stockpiled to treat susceptible individuals once a biological weapon has been identified.

Non-specific immunostimulation

Here the idea is to boost the general activity of the immune system, or some part of it, without reference to any particular antigen. Some ways of doing this make excellent immunological sense—the administration of cytokines, for example. Several of these are beginning to be used clinically, IFNα being the leader because of its proven value in certain chronic viral infections (and also some tumours). IL-2 and IFNγ are also the subject of clinical trials, mostly for chronic intracellular infections such as leprosy and leishmaniasis. At the opposite extreme are some remedies that seem to belong more to 'fringe' medicine, though of course this does not mean they do not work; examples are ginseng and the Chinese herbal mixtures that cause remissions in otherwise untreatable eczema. Western scientists are finally showing interest in the immunological basis of these effects.

28 Control of infectious disease: chemotherapy

The idea of using chemicals to kill microbes goes back to the discovery by Paul Ehrlich (*c.* 1900) that, because of differences in the metabolism of pathogens (mainly protozoa) and man, certain compounds could damage one but not the other. Ehrlich baptized this 'selective toxicity'. Chemical substances are used at four levels for this purpose:

(1) *disinfectants*, which kill microbes but may also damage human tissues, e.g. hypochlorite (bleach);

(2) *antiseptics*, which kill microbes but are safe in contact with human tissues, e.g. iodine in alcohol;

(3) *chemotherapy*, a general term for the treatment of infection with any kind of chemical or antibiotic given systemically;

(4) *antibiotics*, substances produced by a microorganism that damage another microorganism, e.g. penicillin; however, the term is generally applied to synthetic substances too, e.g. sulphonamides.

Chemotherapy has been extremely successful against many bacteria, because their procaryotic structure offers several targets absent from eucaryotic cells (see Fig. 3.1). Antiviral chemotherapy is on the whole less effective (see later). Fortunately the opposite is true for vaccines, which are in general more effective against viruses than bacteria (see Chapter 27). It is much more difficult to devise drugs that attack eucaryotic organisms such as fungi, protozoa, and worms without damaging host cells, and unfortunately there are no human vaccines for eucaryotes either.

Antibacterial agents

These fall into five main categories, depending on the point of action (Table 28.1). The pioneer modern antibacterials were the synthetic azo-dye sulphanilamide (1935) and the true antibiotics penicillin, made by the fungus *Penicillium*, discovered by Fleming in 1929 and first used in 1940, and streptomycin (1944), made by the filamentous bacterium *Streptomyces* and used mainly for tuberculosis. Earlier metal-based drugs, such as the arsenical salvarsan used for syphilis, were

Table 28.1 Some widely used antibacterial drugs, showing their site of action. The term 'broad spectrum' usually implies activity against Gram-positive and Gram-negative bacteria, and often *Chlamydia*, *Rickettsia*, etc. as well

Site of action	Examples	Principal uses
Cell wall peptidoglycan synthesis	β lactams penicillins cephalosporins Glycopeptides vancomycin	Gram + bacteria Gram – bacteria Gram + bacteria
Inner cell membranes	Polymyxins	Gram – bacteria
Protein synthesis	Aminoglycosides streptomycin gentamycin Tetracycline Macrolides erythromycin Chloramphenicol Clindamycin	Tuberculosis Gram – bacteria Broad spectrum Gram + bacteria Broad spectrum Gram + bacteria
Nucleic acid synthesis	Sulphonamides Trimethoprim Rifampicin	Gram – bacteria Gram – bacteria Tuberculosis
DNA	Metronidazole	Anaerobic bacteria
Gyrase	Quinolones ciprofloxacin	Gram –; atypical bacteria
Unknown (mycolic acid synthesis?)	Isoniazid Dapsone	Tuberculosis Leprosy

extremely toxic, but drugs containing arsenic or antimony are still used against some protozoa (see below). Antibiotic research and production proceeds at an ever-increasing pace; about 5000 antibiotics are known, and it is said that about 300 are discovered each year though only about 100 are in common use. It was while screening the fungus *Tolypocladeium inflatium* for antibiotic activity that the dramatically immunosuppressive drug cyclosporin was discovered (1976).

Antibiotic resistance

Considering the ability of microorganisms to elude the immune system by mutation (see Chapter 21) one might expect that they could also develop resistance to chemotherapy, though most people were surprised at how fast this can occur after a new drug is introduced. Gonococci became resistant to sulphonamides within 10 years, and the same happened even faster with staphylococci and penicillin. The explanation is that mutations in the genes for resistance occur spontaneously, and are simply selected out—in other words the bacteria *adapted* to antibiotics in just the same way as the B and T lymphocytes adapt to foreign antigens. Indeed it was while contemplating antibiotic resistance that Jerne, Lederberg, and Burnet worked their way towards the clonal selection theory (see Fig.15.4).

The mechanism is not always the same, however; antibiotic resistance can develop at several levels, ranging from single point mutations to the transfer of whole sets of genes on plasmids or transposons (Table 28.2). As an example, resistance to anti-tuberculous drugs is mainly due to mutation, so it can occur in an individual at any time; the use of 3–4 different drugs together is an attempt to avoid the risk of multiple resistance emerging. On the other hand resistance of *Staphylococcus aureus* to penicillin involves plasmid transfer, and can only be acquired from another individual, which is why it is so common in hospitals. The molecular basis for this resistance, a fascinating battle between microbe and drug for possession of essential components of cell wall synthesis, is illustrated in Fig. 28.1.

Table 28.2 Resistance to antibiotics can be achieved in several ways

Genetic basis	Mode of action	Resistance against
Chromosomal (mutation)	Alteration of target of antibiotic, e.g.	
	ribosome	Streptomycin
	surface permeability	Penicillin
	RNA polymerase	Rifampicin
	membranes	Polymyxin
Plasmid (R factor)	Induction of enzymes that inactivate antibiotic	*Tetracycline *Chloramphenicol *Streptomycin *Sulphonamides Trimethoprim
	β lactamases	Penicillin
	Glycopeptide-binding block	Vancomycin
	Alteration of RNA target	**Erythromycin **Clindamycin **Lincomycin
	Alteration of target enzyme	Sulphonamides Trimethoprim
Transposons	As above, may act in chromosome or plasmid	Tetracycline

The location of several resistance genes on plasmids or transposons allows the very rapid spread of resistance throughout populations of bacteria. *, ** Resistance to these groups of antibiotics is often carried on the same plasmid. Note that antibiotic resistance genes are widely used by molecular biologists to enable a desired population of mutant bacteria to be selected in the laboratory.

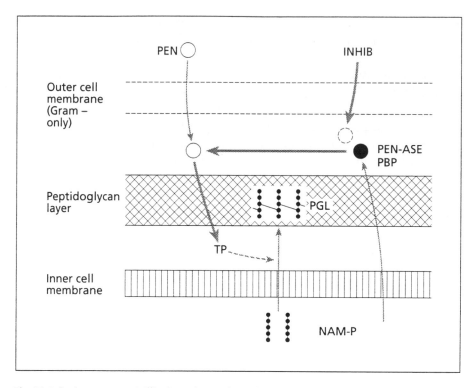

Fig. 28.1 Resistance to penicillin depends mainly on the production by the bacteria of enzymes that destroy the penicillin ring. NAM-P, N-acetyl muramic acid–peptide units; TP, transpeptidases, which join these together, and which are destroyed by penicillin (PEN); PGL, peptidoglycan, the major cell-wall strengthening material; PEN-ASE bacterial penicillinases. Many such enzymes exist, some being more active against penicillins and others being more active against cephalosporins; as a group they are referred to as β-lactamases, and there are also other penicillin-binding proteins (PBP). One possible counter-attack is to use competitive inhibitors (INHIB) of the bacterial enzymes, such as clavulanic acid.

Biofilms and resistance

A biofilm is a bacterial community growing on a surface and enclosed in a poly-saccharide matrix and this, rather than floating free in a laboratory test tube, is how pathogenic bacteria grow in 'real life'. Mucous membranes, teeth, and sur-gically implanted materials are major sites, and it has been found that bacteria in a biofilm can be up to 1000 times more resistant to antibiotics than those grow-ing free. This is partly due to the matrix itself, but also to the fact that in large colonies bacteria do not replicate so fast, and to other less well understood changes. There is some evidence that innate immune mechanisms (e.g. iron depletion by lactoferrin from polymorphs) can inhibit biofilm formation.

Bacterial interference: the normal flora

Another aspect of 'real life' bacterial infection is the existence of enormous num-bers of non-pathogenic bacteria, also growing as biofilms, notably in the gut—

which may contain up to 10^{14} organisms of 500 different species, mostly harmless *commensals* competing with pathogens for space and nutrients. Some may be actively beneficial, for example the lactobacilli which are thought to keep down pathogens, notably *Candida*, in the gut, vagina, mouth, etc. Over-zealous antibiotic treatment, by killing these, may allow pathogens to take over. Attempts have been made to deliberately colonize mucous surfaces with *Lactobacillus* and other 'good' or *probiotic* bacteria.

Toxicity

The other problem with antibiotics, as with all drugs, is toxicity. This can be due to the drug directly, or to an immune response against it. In fact, drugs are a major cause of hypersensitivity reactions, and a substantial number of these are due to antibiotics (Table 28.3). A third possibility is that the simultaneous destruction of many pathogens may release enough material to induce strong

Table 28.3 Anti-microbial drugs account for a large proportion of drug toxicity, which may be direct or secondary to an immune response—usually to the drug bound to some body component, i.e. acting as a *hapten*

Mechanism	Examples	Clinical effects
Direct		
Renal damage	Aminoglycosides	Renal failure
	Amphotericin (antifungal)	Renal failure
Auditory nerve damage	Aminoglycosides	Dizziness, deafness
Bone marrow depression	Chloramphenicol	Infections, bleeding
	Zidovudine (antiviral)	Infections, bleeding
Changed gut flora	Tetracycline	Diarrhoea
Deposition in teeth	Tetracycline	Staining (children)
Hypersensitivity		
Type I (allergic)	*Penicillin ⎫ Sulphonamides ⎭	Rashes *Anaphylaxis
Type II (cytotoxic)	Penicillin ⎫ Sulphonamides ⎭	Haemolytic anaemia (autoimmune)
Type III (immune complexes)	Penicillin ⎫ Sulphonamides ⎭	Erythema Nephritis
Type IV (cell-mediated)	Penicillin ⎫ Sulphonamides ⎬ Streptomycin ⎭	Contact dermatitis

*Hypersensitivity to penicillin is the commonest cause of anaphylaxis—except perhaps among bee-keepers!

inflammatory reactions; examples are syphilis, relapsing fever, Lyme disease, tuberculosis, and African trypanosomiasis.

Antiviral drugs

With viruses, the problem is that many of the steps in viral replication are provided by the host cell itself, and cannot be blocked without killing the cell. One solution is that adopted by the immune system: kill both virus and cell, which is what NK cells and cytotoxic cells do (see Chapters 11 and 19). However, nature, by evolving the *interferons*, has shown that specific antiviral activity is a possibility, and a few drugs are now available that exploit small differences between host and viral metabolism, usually at the enzyme level (Table 28.4). In general, however, vaccines have proved more useful against viruses than drugs have; moreover, some viruses are able to develop resistance.

Drugs against fungi, protozoa, and worms

Most of the effective drugs against these eucaryotic infections display considerable toxicity (side-effects) to their (eucaryotic) animal host, and they have to be used with caution. Tables 28.5–7 list the generally available ones. The story of malaria illustrates some of the problems. The effect of *quinine*, a plant derivative, has been known for over three centuries, and it is still a drug of choice for acute life-threatening malaria, despite its side-effects (which include hypoglycaemia, hypotension, cardiac arrhythmias, and disturbances of hearing and vision).

Table 28.4 Antiviral compounds are not as dramatically effective as most antibacterials, but steady progress is being made

Compound	Site of action	Effective against
Naturally occurring		
Interferon (mainly α)	Viral RNA translation	Hepatitis B (in carriers)
	Viral protein synthesis (plus effects on T and NK cells)	Herpesviruses *Common cold
Synthetic		
Amantidine	Entry into cell	Influenza A
Acyclovir ⎫	DNA polymerase	Herpesviruses
Ganciclovir ⎭		
Zidovudine (AZT)	Reverse transcriptase	Retroviruses (e.g. HIV)
Oreltamivir	Neuraminidase	Influenza A, B

* The proved effectiveness of interferon in preventing colds has not led to clinical use because of high cost and unpleasant side-effects.

Table 28.5 Some drugs in use against fungi; those asterisked are the most effective against severe systemic infection

Drug	Active against	Side-effects
Cell wall inhibitors		
Caspofungin	*Candida, Aspergillus*	Rare
Ergosterol inhibitors (damage cell membrane)		
Terbinafine	Dermatophytes	Nausea, rash
Fluconazole	Yeasts	Nausea, liver damage
Itraconazole	" ; *Aspergillus*	Hepatitis
Voriconazole	Yeasts, moulds, *Aspergillus*	Visual
*Ketoconazole	Dermatophytes, *Candida*	Nausea, hepatitis
*Amphotericin B	Most moulds and yeasts	Renal toxicity
Nystatin	*Candida* (superficial)	Skin staining
Inhibitors of mitosis		
Griseofulvin	Dermatophytes	Nausea, visual
Inhibitors of protein synthesis		
Flucytosin	*Candida, Cryptococcus*	Neutropenia, jaundice

Table 28.6 Some drugs used against protozoal infections

Disease	Drug/regime	Comments
Malaria		
Liver stage	Primaquine/oral	
Blood stage	Chloroquine/oral	Resistance common
	Artemisinin derivatives	Resistance rare
Acute, cerebral	Quinine IM/IV	Severe toxicity
Leishmaniasis	Antimonials; pentamidine	Severe toxicity
	Amphotericin B	" "
Sleeping sickness	Suramin; pentamidine	" "
	Melarsoprol	" (CNS)
Chagas' disease	Nifurtimox; benznidazone	" "
Toxoplasmosis	Pentamidine; pyrimethamine	" "
Amoebiasis		
Intestinal	Diloxanide	
Systemic; abscess	Metronidazole	
Giardiasis	Metronidazole; tinidazole	
Cryptosporidiosis	Spiramycin; pyrimethamine; nitazoximide	
Trichomoniasis	Metronidazole; tinidazole	

Table 28.7 Some drugs used against helminth infections

Disease	Drug/regime
Flukes	
Schistosomiasis	Praziquantel; oxamniquine
Fascioliasis	Triclabendazole
Roundworms	
Filariasis	*Ivermectin; diethylcarbamizine; albendazole
Intestinal	Mebendazole; albendazole; levamisole
Trichinosis	Mebendazole; thiabendazole
Tapeworms	
Taenia	Praziquantel; niclosamide
Hydatid	Albendazole

* often used in combination

Choloroquine, a more practical drug for preventive use requiring less frequent dosage, was introduced in the 1940s, but between 1960 and 1990 chloroquine resistance emerged and spread round the world, and though new antimalarials are regularly produced, the parasites usually appear to be able to keep one step ahead. Recently, however, derivatives of a traditional Chinese herb, *artemisia*, have shown great promise. It is curious that few plant products other than the two major antimalarials are medically established for the treatment of infection. Another success story is the discovery of two important new anti-helminthics (anti-worm drugs), *praziquantel* and *ivermectin*, which exploit differences in neuromuscular action between worm and host.

Chemotherapy and the immune system

The role of immunity in drug toxicity has already been mentioned. Many anti-microbial agents kill their target directly, but others appears to need some degree of help from the immune system. As a result immunocompromised patients may need lifelong treatment for infections that would require only a short course of treatment in normal individuals. For example, pentostam (antimony sodium gluconate) is not effective against leishmaniasis in the absence of a T-cell response. The powerful immunosuppressive effect of the otherwise promising antibiotic cyclosporin has already been mentioned. Some drugs accumulate in macrophages, making them more effective against intracellular pathogens. The same effect may be achieved by encapsulating them in lipid vesicles—an example being liposomal amphotericin B. Finally, some antibiotics are themselves immunostimulatory.

29 Control of infectious disease: public health measures

A concern for the health of others could be considered as one of the hallmarks of a civilized society, and for centuries before the invention of vaccines or antibiotics societies have investigated ways of limiting infectious disease. In the previous two chapters we described how tuberculosis can be largely controlled both by vaccination and by chemotherapy, yet a careful study of the incidence of the disease in England and Wales shows the surprising fact that the incidence, particularly in younger people, had already fallen by about a third between 1850 and 1900—before either vaccine or drug treatment had started. This improvement was due to the general improvement in health that accompanied better nutrition and food handling, better housing and housing regulations, stronger legislation, and a more enlightened attitude to social problems, which continued throughout the 20th century, helped in the case of *M. bovis* by Pasteur's heating technique (Fig. 29.1). The elimination of cholera in Europe and the US, and its reduction elsewhere, owed far more to proper separation of sewage and drinking water than to the not very effective vaccine. Some other success stories that have nothing to do with vaccines or drugs are listed in Table 29.1.

Some of the above measures imply prolonged or continuous efforts and a certain restriction of normal human activity, with a tendency to relax these as they are seen to take effect and disease begins to retreat. Often a degree of self-sacrifice is required; for instance not everybody with a cold or influenza is prepared to stay at home or wear a mask, though this would clearly benefit others. The famous Typhoid Mary, a New York cook who was a typhoid carrier, repeatedly refused to abandon cooking, even in the face of a prison sentence. Nurses with virulent staphylococci in their noses are taken off duty and treated. Specially vigorous control measures are needed in hospitals since (1) conditions are unusually crowded, with hundreds of person–person contacts per day, (2) patients frequently bring infection in with them, (3) antibiotic-resistant and opportunist infections are more common in hospitals than in the community as a whole, and (4) many patients will be relatively immunodeficient because of their disease or surgery. Also to be considered, of course, is the psychological effect of catching a serious disease in hospital.

By contrast vaccines and antibiotics, apart from occasional side-effects, normally benefit the individual without any inconvenience—although here, too, there are ethical issues; for example the question whether patients with multiple

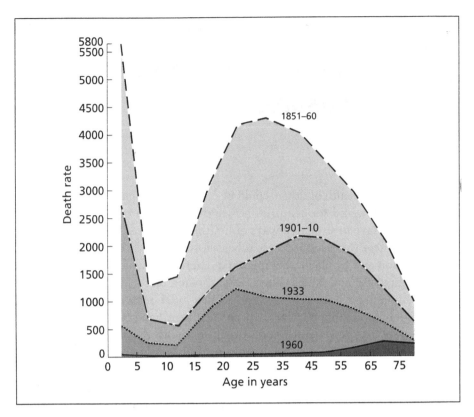

Fig. 29.1 Death rates per million from tuberculosis (all forms), England and Wales, showing the changing pattern of infection. Note that chemotherapy was not introduced until 1944, while the BCG vaccine, though produced in the 1920s, was not widely used until the 1950s, yet the disease had already declined by about 80%, particularly in the younger age group.

drug-resistant infections should be isolated and/or obliged to take appropriate antibiotics, and whether vaccination should be compulsory.

Note that even when a vaccine has been developed and introduced, public health organizations are still an important element in disease control. The numbers vaccinated, the numbers who seroconvert, and the numbers who develop disease will all have to be accurately monitored. Moreover if the vaccine fails and is abandoned, it is vital for the alternative means of disease control to continue being enforced.

Animals without pathogens?

Continuous advances in vaccine and antibiotic technology, combined with ever more draconian public health control of food, water, vectors, etc., might tempt the unwary to dream of a world without pathogens. This seems an extremely un-

Table 29.1 Some examples of attempted disease control through public health measures

Disease/organism	How controlled
Leprosy (Middle Ages)	Quarantine of cases (in lazarettos)
"	Isolation of cases (in leprosaria)
Cholera (London, 1855)	Identification of contaminated water source
Typhoid	Water purification; quarantine of cases
Legionella	Maintenance of air-conditioning cooling systems
Hospital staphylococci	Screening of possible carriers (nurses, etc.)
HIV, hepatitis B, malaria	Screening of blood donors
Tuberculosis (bovine)	Heating of milk (pasteurization)
Brucellosis	" "
Sexually transmitted diseases	Advice, condoms
Malaria (Rome, 1935)	Draining of marshes where mosquito vector breeds
Malaria (tropical)	Killing of mosquitoes by DDT, etc.
"	Insecticide-impregnated mosquito nets
" (non-tropical)	Fumigation of aircraft
Plague; typhus	Control of rat reservoir/insect vector
Rabies	Killing of rabid dogs
Hydatid disease	Reduced contact with dog reservoir
Schistosomiasis (China)	Draining of ditches where snail vector breeds
" (Africa, S. America)	Education of danger of barefoot paddling
Onchocerciasis	Spraying insecticide on rivers to kill fly vector

likely prospect. In the first place, *bacteria* appear in general to be beneficial to higher animals; no less a scientist than Pasteur stated that 'microbes are essential for normal life'. He was certainly right in the sense that animals deprived of their normal flora—particularly that of the intestine—or born and raised in the total absence of any form of microbe, show reductions in weight, metabolic rate, cardiac output, etc. Such 'germ-free' or *gnotobiotic* animals can be kept alive and reasonably healthy, provided they do not become exposed to pathogens, which in practice means very careful and expensive housing and feeding. Indeed, such animals, mainly mice, have been of great value in understanding infection, nutrition, cancer, ageing, and many other areas where host and pathogen normally both make a contribution. However, it is impossible to imagine a way in which the germ-free state could come about or persist naturally, given the limitless reservoir of free-living bacteria, any of which could theoretically become adapted to a parasitic existence and some of which, being newcomers to the human ecosystem, would probably cause pathology.

In fact, it is much easier to imagine a world of microbes without higher animals, which must have existed billions of years ago and could again, if the worst predictions of nuclear Armageddon were ever to come about, because there are bacteria that can survive at extraordinary ranges of temperature (−12°C, 105°C), oxygen concentration (including none), radiation (1–2 megarads, the fatal dose for man being well under 1 kilorad), water and salt concentration, etc. The evolution of higher animals would then, presumably, have to start all over again—a depressing but intriguing thought.

30 Viral and prion disease and immunity

The general features of viruses and prions are discussed in Chapters 2 and 7, and Chapters 10–25 describe the immune mechanisms that combat them. During their intracellular phase, viruses are generally most efficiently dealt with by interferon, NK cells, and cytotoxic T cells, while when spreading from cell to cell they become susceptible to antibody (Fig. 30.1). Most viruses have well-developed *escape mechanisms*, they frequently cause *immunopathology*, and some are *opportunists*. Fortunately, there are some excellent antiviral *vaccines*. In this chapter we will survey the individual features of the common virus infections, considered from a clinical, pathological, and immunological, rather than a taxonomic, viewpoint.

The common childhood viruses

Measles, mumps, and rubella are similar in being spread by the respiratory route and infecting a high proportion of contacts, measles especially, with prominent skin rashes. Since there is only one antigenic type of each, the immunity following recovery is virtually lifelong. *Measles* virus can infect T cells and dendritic cells, and causes a transient immunosuppression, with increased susceptibility to e.g. tuberculosis. As mentioned in Chapter 25, measles can be severe or fatal in malnourished children. *Mumps* is interesting as a rare cause of autoimmune orchitis. *Rubella* is particularly important because of its effect on the growing fetus during the first three months of pregnancy: blindness, deafness, heart defects, and mental retardation occur in up to a quarter of cases (other viruses that can cause congenital malformation are CMV and chickenpox). Attenuated vaccines against measles, mumps, and rubella (the MMR vaccine) are highly effective, and the recent 'scare' about a link with autism (not convincingly proved) has already led to a decreased uptake, and some resurgence of measles has already occurred, which is unfortunate because measles is considered as a possible candidate for complete eradication. The herpesvirus HHV3 *(varicella-zoster*; *VZV)* also gives lifelong immunity to the primary disease (chickenpox) but can persist in nerve cells and reappear many years later in the form of shingles (zoster), with painful vesicular skin lesions on the trunk from which

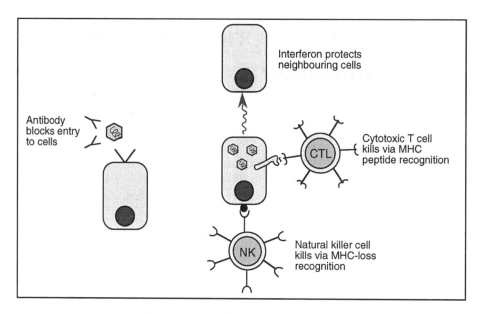

Fig. 30.1 Antiviral immunity; an overview.

susceptible children can catch chickenpox. There is an effective vaccine but its use is not routine. Note that despite its name, chickenpox is quite unrelated to the pox viruses such as *smallpox*—now eradicated.

Skin rashes

While the rash of chickenpox is due to the destruction of cells by the virus, the rashes of measles and rubella appear to be immunopathological and probably T-cell mediated. This is illustrated by the fact that children with T cell deficiency do not develop a measles rash but a fatal systemic infection.

The common cold

Colds can be caused by a variety of viruses, notably rhinovirus, coronavirus, Coxsackie virus, and echovirus. Since there are from 20 to 100 antigenic types of each, one can suffer hundreds of colds without meeting the same type twice, so that in effect there is no useful immunity following recovery and very little prospect of a vaccine. Fortunately most colds are short-lived, mainly due to the local activity of interferon and NK cells, and simple anticongestants will relieve most of the symptoms. It has been shown that intranasal interferon α will prevent most colds—if administered before the virus!

Influenza

Of the three types of influenza (A, B, and C), influenza A is the most serious, because of the *antigenic variation* (see Chapter 21) that affects its H and N surface antigens, preventing the build-up of B and T cell memory. Minor variants produced by accumulated mutations (antigenic *drift*) are responsible for the fact that each year's outbreak is antigenically different, and for the major epidemics that occur every decade or so. The much larger antigenic *shifts* that occur when the human virus exchanges RNA with one from a bird (the recombination usually occurring in pigs, which are susceptible to both bird and human flu) give rise to massive pandemics like the one that followed the First World War, killing more people than the war itself. An inactivated *vaccine* is nowadays given to those in the high-risk category (the elderly, nurses, doctors, cardiac, diabetic, immunodeficient patients, etc.), but it has to be made afresh every year because of antigenic drift. A stable living vaccine has not so far been achieved.

Other respiratory viruses

Most of the viruses affecting the nose and throat can spread to the bronchi and lungs. *Respiratory syncytial virus* (RSV) is a very common cause of bronchiolitis and pneumonia in young children. A killed vaccine was tried, but caused enhanced disease with pulmonary essinophilia. The first measles vaccine also increased pathology due to production of non-neutralizing antibodies resulting in immune complex (Type III) hypersensitivity.

Glandular fever

This unpleasant disease bristles with interesting immunology. It is caused by the herpesvirus HHV4, usually called EBV after its discoverers (Epstein and Barr, in 1964), and is also known as *infectious mononucleosis* because of the 'atypical monocytes' seen in the blood. These are in fact cytotoxic T lymphocytes directed against the EBV-infected cells, which are mainly B lymphocytes and the pharyngeal mucosa—a clear-cut example of useful CD8 T cell immunity (see Chapter 19). Because it is easily spread by saliva and affects mainly teenagers, it is sometimes called 'kissing disease'. Recovery is the rule, but can take several weeks; very rarely the disease can be acutely fatal or become chronic. In tropical countries EBV infection is more likely to occur unnoticed in childhood, and glandular fever is rare. Instead, in conjunction with repeated malaria infection, EBV can cause Burkitt's lymphoma, a B-cell tumour mainly of the jaw. In the Far East EBV is involved in nasopharyngeal carcinoma, and in AIDS patients it can give rise to B cell tumours in the brain. Finally, EBV has also been thought by some to be responsible for a proportion of cases of the mysterious *chronic fatigue syndrome*.

Other herpesviruses

The herpes simplex viruses HSV1 and HSV2 cause cold sores and genital herpes, and like varicella they can persist in nerve cells and reappear as painful demarcated skin lesions. There is no vaccine but prolonged treatment with *acyclovir* is very effective. Cytomegalovirus (CMV or HHV5), mainly important as an opportunist, causes severe pneumonitis in AIDS patients and in those immunosuppressed for bone marrow transplantation. HHV8 is the cause of Kaposi's sarcoma in AIDS patients.

Poliomyelitis

This once feared paralytic enterovirus disease is another candidate for eventual elimination, thanks to two highly effective vaccines: inactivated (Salk, 1954) and attenuated (Sabin, 1957), each of which still has its staunch supporters (see Chapter 27).

Other enteroviruses

Echovirus and Coxsackie virus have been mentioned as causes of colds; they can also, like polio, cause meningitis. *Hepatitis A* is discussed below. Note that the name *enterovirus* describes the site of spread (oral–faecal) and replication, rather than the site of infection. In fact most viral diarrhoea is caused by the unrelated *rotaviruses*.

Hepatitis

There are at least five hepatitis viruses, giving a similar clinical pattern but with different outcomes. *Hepatitis A* is normally a self-limiting infection. There is a good vaccine, recommended for travellers to the tropics; passively injected pooled immunoglobulin also gives good short-term protection. *Hepatitis B* is more serious. Normally eliminated, mainly by cytotoxic T cells that kill the infected liver cells, it can persist in about 10% of patients, who become *carriers*, able to infect others. Further complications are chronic active hepatitis, cirrhosis, and liver carcinoma. Fortunately there is a highly effective vaccine—the first to be produced by recombinant DNA technology. *Hepatitis C* is similar but is even more likely to lead to chronic active hepatitis and cirrhosis.

Rabies

This virus is celebrated for Pasteur's extraordinarily lucky vaccine experiment (see Tutorial 4). Rabies is unusual in that the virus travels slowly along nerves, taking weeks to get from the site of infection (usually a dog bite) to the brain, where it infects and damages neurones (encephalitis). This allows time for both passive antiserum and active vaccination to give protection. Other viral causes of encephalitis include herpesviruses, mumps, togavirus, and HIV.

Viral zoonoses

In addition to rabies, some of the most acutely fatal viral diseases are derived from animal hosts, in which they are usually much milder infections. *Lassa* fever (from African bush rats), *Hanta* virus (from American and Scandinavian rodents), and *Marburg* and *Ebola* fever (from as yet unidentified African animals) are characterized by severe haemorrhages into the skin and internal organs.

Yellow fever and dengue

These viral haemorrhagic viruses are unusual in being spread by mosquitoes. Bleeding defects are a major feature and in dengue a particularly severe haemorrhagic shock syndrome can occur, in which non-neutralizing antibodies enhance the entry of the virus into monocytes, triggering the release of inflammatory cytokines. The very effective attenuated yellow fever vaccine is remarkable in having remained stable since 1937. There is no effective dengue vaccine yet.

Papilloma viruses

Ten of the more than 70 types of human papilloma viruses are associated with various kinds of warts, and others with cancer of the cervix and, more rarely, penis, anus, and larynx.

Retroviruses

HIV is discussed in Chapter 25. The only other retroviruses of significance to man are the *human T cell lymphotropic viruses* HTLV-1 and HTLV-2. HTLV-1 causes T cell leukaemia and lymphoma, but only in about 1% of infected people. It appears to promote the growth of T cells by stimulating IL-15.

Prion diseases (transmissible spongiform encephalopathies; TSE)

The first prion disease to be clearly shown to be infectious was *kuru*, a neurological condition seen only among the Fore people of New Guinea and transmitted by ritual eating of the brains of ancestors. Very much as with BSE in cattle, the disease gradually died out as this practice was abandoned. The main symptom was a Parkinsonian tremor, indicating involvement of the cerebellum. Shortly after, *Creutzfeldt–Jakob disease* (CJD) was also shown to be transmissible (see Chapter 7 for the history). In this condition, after an incubation period of many years, dementia and ataxia are the commonest presenting symptoms, usually fatal within a year. The main pathological finding is spongiform vacuolation in the cerebral cortex. Four varieties are currently recognized (see Table 30.1).

Table 30.1 Human prion diseases and their transmission

Iatrogenic (iCJD)	Contamination of growth hormone, dura mater grafts, corneal grafts, surgical instruments
Familial (fCJD)	Germ-line mutation in PrP gene (more than 20 known)
Sporadic (sCJD)	Somatic mutation in PrP gene; transmission?
New variant (vCJD)	Contaminated beef from BSE cattle
Kuru	Cannibalism

31 Bacterial disease and immunity

First, re-read Chapter 3 to remind yourself of the key properties of bacteria and the all-important distinction between extracellular and intracellular habitat. In general, extracellular bacteria are dealt with by the combination antibody + complement + phagocytic cells, while intracellular ones (usually resident in macrophages) depend largely on T cells + cytokines such as IFNγ for their control.

Staphylococcal infection

These Gram-positive extracellular bacteria, transmitted by contact and airborne droplets, are the cause of most pyogenic (pus-forming) infections of the skin and soft tissues, sometimes spreading to lungs and bone. Healthy nasal carriers of *Staphylococcus aureus* are a major source of infection, especially in hospitals. Many strains produce numerous exotoxins, with both local effects (tissue destruction, coagulation of serum, abscess formation) and more distant ones (food poisoning, toxic shock). Other virulence factors include the anti-phagocytic capsule and the IgG-neutralizing Protein A. Deficiencies of neutrophil function (see Chapter 14) predispose to severe chronic staphylococcal infections. Penicillin was originally effective but most staphylococci, particularly in hospitals, are now resistant, these being usually referred to as MRSA (methicillin-resistant *S. aureus*); some are now resistant to the newer antibiotic vancomycin too. There are no effective anti-staphylococcal vaccines.

Streptococcal infection

Group A streptococci are a common cause of sore throats and, less often, of spreading skin infections (including the 'flesh-eating superbug' beloved of popular journalism). Complications include scarlet fever (due to an erythrogenic exotoxin), rheumatic fever, myocarditis (an autoimmune consequence of cross-reaction between bacterial and myocardial antigens), and glomerulonephritis (an immune-complex-mediated hypersensitivity reaction). *Streptococcus pneumoniae* (formerly the pneumococcus), a major cause of lobar pneumonia and meningitis, has an anti-phagocytic capsule, but IgG antibody to capsular polysaccharides allows phagocytosis and destruction of the organisms by neutrophils; the current vaccine consists of about 50 different strain-specific capsular polysaccharide variants. *S. mutans* is a major cause of dental caries and experimental vaccines have been tried in monkeys. Otherwise there are no effective anti-streptococcal vaccines. *S. faecalis*, an important cause of postoperative septicaemia, has been reclassified as *Enterococcus*.

Anthrax

Mainly a disease of farm animals and farmers, anthrax has achieved notoriety as a possible weapon of biological warfare. A major feature is that spores can persist for decades in the environment. It begins as an ulcerating skin lesion which may proceed to septicaemia and death from the effects of the exotoxin. There is a good attenuated vaccine and high-dose penicillin is also effective.

Clostridial infections

Clostridia are soil-dwellers, surviving adverse conditions by forming spores. Their pathological effects are due to exotoxins (see Chapter 8) with effects on nerve-muscle transmission (*Clostridium tetani*: tetanus; *C. botulinum*: botulism) and tissue destruction in deep wounds (*C. perfringens*: gas gangrene). Treatment is by passive immunization with antitoxin, and there is an effective toxoid vaccine against tetanus, introduced during the early months of World War I and nowadays given as a triple vaccine together with diphtheria toxoid and killed *Bordetella pertussis* (see below).

Diphtheria

Destruction of pharyngeal epithelium by the exotoxin of *Corynebacterium diphtheriae* gives rise to a 'false membrane' which can cause respiratory obstruction. Sometimes there is also damage to the heart and nervous system. The disease is now rare thanks to the universal use of the toxoid vaccine (see above). Of the many other corynebacteria, *C. jeikeium* is emerging as an important opportunist.

Listeriosis

Listeria monocytogenes, usually acquired from animals via uncooked food, is an opportunist—an important cause of meningitis in immunodeficient patients and, since it is transmitted across the placenta, the newborn. The organism is mainly intracellular, spreading from macrophage to macrophage by a form of budding that allows it to remain totally concealed. T_H1 cells, cytotoxic T cells, and NK cells are all thought to play a part in immunity, both via activation of macrophages (by IFNγ) and by direct cytotoxicity. No vaccine is available.

Mycobacteria I: tuberculosis (TB)

The most important mycobacterial infection and one of the world's major health problems. Spread by droplet (mainly from coughs), *Mycobacterium tuberculosis* is the classic example of a bacterium capable of surviving for long periods in macrophages, which enables it to cause chronic and often lifelong infections. Being aerobic, it prefers the well-oxygenated parts of the lung, but can spread to almost any other organ if cell-mediated immunity becomes inadequate, and can also survive at low oxygen concentrations in granulomas. This capacity for survival makes it a major problem in undernourished or immunodeficient patients. In nineteenth-century Britain tuberculosis was responsible for about 20% of deaths, and the AIDS epidemic has caused a resurgence of the disease in the tropics.

The pathology, based on tissue necrosis and granuloma formation, is also due to cell-mediated mechanisms (Type IV; see Chapter 22). Broadly speaking, T_H1 cells, secreting IFNγ, are beneficial, and T_H2 cells (and antibody) useless or harmful, but all the elements in the balance between health and disease are not fully understood. A positive Mantoux (delayed hypersensitivity) skin test denotes previous exposure but does not guarantee immunity. The attenuated vaccine (BCG) is widely used but varies markedly in its effectiveness in different parts of the world. Chemotherapy requires combinations of up to three drugs, maintained for several months. *M. bovis* was a cause of human TB before pasteurization of milk; *M. avium intracellulare* has emerged as an important pathogen in AIDS patients.

Mycobacteria II: leprosy

M. leprae resembles *M. tuberculosis* in many ways but is restricted to skin and superficial tissues, causing terrible deformities to the face and extremities. It is the classic example of the balance or 'spectrum' between T_H1 (cell-mediated) and T_H2 (antibody-mediated) immunity. A predominantly T_H1 response results in killing of the bacteria with scarring and destruction of peripheral nerves (tuberculoid leprosy); a predominantly T_H2 pattern leads to uncontrolled growth of bacteria in superficial tissues (lepromatous leprosy); several intermediate stages are recognized and patients may move from one to another as a result of treatment. The immune mechanisms by which about a third of infected individuals control the disease without symptoms are not understood. The BCG vaccine gives some protection, but the main hope for elimination is by combination chemotherapy (dapsone, rifampin, plus one other drug).

Meningococcal meningitis

Neisseria meningitidis (the meningococcus) is a Gram-negative capsulated diplococcus carried in the nasopharynx of some 20% of healthy people, which for ill-understood reasons can occasionally spread to the meninges (meningitis) or the blood (septicaemia). Based on the polysaccharide capsular antigens, three serotypes are recognized (A, B, C), of which B is the commonest cause of disease. Unfortunately the type B polysaccharide is the least immunogenic, since it is mainly sialic acid; as a result there are good polysaccharide vaccines against A and C but not B. Unlike most other bacteria, *Neisseria* are largely eliminated by antibody plus the lytic complement pathway, so people deficient in C5–9 are more susceptible. Meningococcal septicaemia is a dangerous complication, associated with a skin rash, vascular collapse, and acute renal and adrenal failure; excessive production of cytokines, especially TNF, is thought to be responsible.

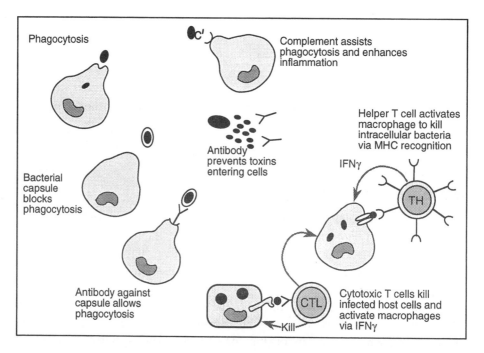

Fig. 31.1 Antibacterial immunity: an overview.

Gonorrhoea

Neisseria gonorrhoeae (the gonococcus) resembles *N. meningitidis* in susceptibility to complement lysis and the use of pili—in this case to attach to the genito-urinary mucosa. An anti-phagocytic capsule, two pore-forming proteins, and an IgA-destroying enzyme complete a formidable list of virulence factors. Infection is usually limited to the genito-urinary tract, with rare systemic complications (arthritis, endocarditis). There is no vaccine but a variety of antibiotics are effective.

Enteric infections

The enterobacteria group includes a number of organisms spread by the oral–faecal route, capable of causing diarrhoea and/or urinary infection with occasional systemic spread. Some, such as *Proteus* and *Klebsiella*, are part of the normal gut flora, while *Salmonella* and *Shigella* are not. Some strains of *Escherichia coli* occur normally, while others are enterotoxic (ETEC), enteropathogenic (EPEC), invasive (EIEC), or haemorrhagic (EHEC, which includes the notorious O157 strain). *Salmonella typhi*, the cause of typhoid fever, survives within macrophages and is disseminated to lymph nodes and, via the bloodstream, to other organs. Without treatment about 15% of patients die, and following recovery up to 3% continue to excrete the organisms; these *carriers* are responsible for fresh outbreaks. The original killed typhoid vaccine was unpleasant (due to the endotoxin content) and only partly effective; more recent candidates are (1) an attenuated organism with deletion of genes needed for long-term survival (GalE, AroA); and (2) a purified capsular polysaccharide, the Vi (virulence) antigen. Vaccines against *Shigella* and *E.coli* are still at the experimental stage.

Plague

Yersinia pestis, a mild infection in rats transmitted by fleas, periodically causes human epidemics, in which either the bubonic (lymph node) or the pneumonic form may predominate. Both carry a high mortality, but survivors are immune to reinfection and there is a fairly effective killed vaccine. Tetracycline gives good prophylactic protection.

Pseudomonas and *Burkholderia*

P. aeruginosa has become important as an opportunist infection of the lungs in patients with cystic fibrosis. *B. (formerly P.) mallei* and *pseudomallei*, have been proposed as potential agents of biological warfare, and the latter causes septi-caemía in SE Asia.

Cholera

Vibrio cholerae gives rise to the characteristic rapid watery diarrhoea ('rice water stool') of cholera by secreting a toxin that raises cAMP levels in intestinal ep-ithelial cells, causing them to lose water and electrolytes—up to a litre per hour. Thus the patient, if untreated, dies of dehydration. The widely used killed vac-cine is now considered to be fairly ineffective and experimental approaches are directed at the toxin. To be effective, an anti-toxin vaccine would have to induce high levels of IgA in the intestine.

Campylobacter and *Helicobacter* infection

C. jejuni and *H. pylori* (formerly known as *C. pylori*) are common causes of di-arrhoea and gastritis, respectively. *H. pylori* survives in the highly acid environ-ment of the stomach by producing urease which breaks down urea to ammonia. The resulting inflammation is thought to underlie not only gastric and duodenal ulcers but also gastric carcinoma. Immunity may contribute to these through the local production of cytokines and the attraction and activation of neutrophils.

Brucellosis

Normally an infection of animals (*Brucella abortus*: cattle; *B. melitensis*: sheep and goats; *B. suis*: pigs), *Brucella* infect man by contact or food contamination (e.g. milk). An undulant pattern of fever results, the organism residing and spreading in macrophages. Diagnosis is by blood culture, and treatment is by an-tibiotics. Though there is an attenuated vaccine for animals, it has not been used in man. Since very few organisms are needed for infection, laboratory-acquired infection is a possibility.

Haemophilus infection

H. influenzae is normally present in the throat, but the capsulated Type b ('Hib') may spread to the lungs and/or the meninges. *Haemophilus* meningitis is com-monest in children from about 6 months to 3 years old, since during this age pe-riod maternally transmitted antibody has waned and they do not yet produce their own IgG antibody against the capsular polysaccharide. Infections of the lungs, bronchi, sinuses, middle ear, and epiglottis are usually secondary to virus infection. A polysaccharide vaccine, usually conjugated to a protein 'carrier', produces excellent protection. Another species of *Haemophilus*, *H. ducreyi*, causes genital 'soft chancre'.

Pertussis

Bordetella pertussis causes the childhood disease pertussis, or whooping cough. The bacterium is rich in virulence factors, including an endotoxin, an exotoxin, a toxin that damages phagocytes, and another that inhibits the beating of cilia in the bronchi and trachea—thus arresting the 'muco-ciliary escalator'. There is an effective killed vaccine, given with tetanus and diphtheria toxoids, but it has been suspected of dangerous side-effects, notably convulsions and brain damage, probably due to the endotoxin. As a result, during the 1970s many parents refused the vaccine and in the winter of 1978–79 the death-rate from whooping cough rose dramatically. Several new approaches are under trial, based on either inactivated toxins or genetically modified avirulent whole bacteria.

Legionellosis

Only discovered in 1976, the intracellular bacillus *Legionella pneumophilia* grows in water from industrial cooling towers, hot water, and air conditioning systems, from which it is spread by aerosol. Legionnaire's disease presents as an 'atypical' pneumonia; the name *atypical* derives from its failure to respond to penicillin as 'classic' pneumococcal pneumonia does and the name of the disease refers to a convention of the American Legion where the first outbreak occurred. A rare complication is encephalitis. There is no vaccine but erythromycin is effective.

Bacteroides

B. fragilis, a normal gut commensal, is a common cause of peritonitis following trauma to the gut or surgery. Treatment is with gentamycin.

Syphilis

Caused by the spirally coiled spirochaete *Treponema pallidum*, syphilis was the major venereal disease before the advent of penicillin. It was much feared because of its slow and inexorable course, often taking 20–30 years to kill the patient from damage to the brain, heart valves, or other organs. The organism induces numerous antibodies, including one that cross-reacts with the normal mammalian phospholipid cardiolipin (the Wasserman reaction), but although about a third of patients recover spontaneously, it is not known what immune response if any is responsible, nor how the bacteria survive in the patients who progress. Early treatments with metals (arsenic, bismuth, mercury) led to the cynical summary of syphilitic infection as 'one night with Venus, a lifetime with Mercury'.

Leptospirosis

Leptospirosis, or Weil's disease, caused by the spiral bacterium *Leptospira interrogans*, is a multi-system zoonosis caught from rats and domestic animals via contaminated food or water. In a small number of cases there may be haemorrhages in the brain, eye, liver, and kidney, leading to liver and/or kidney failure. Penicillin and tetracycline are effective.

Borrelia infection

B. recurrentis, the cause of relapsing fever, a spiral bacterium spread by body lice, was one of the first bacteria in which antigenic variation was shown, allowing it to escape the antibody response, much as influenza and African trypanosomes do (see Chapter 21). *B. burgdorferi* is spread by ticks and causes Lyme disease, a migrating skin rash followed weeks or years later by brain, heart, and joint lesions, possibly autoimmune in origin. Treatment is as for Weil's disease.

Actinomycosis

Actinomyces israeli is often found in dental plaque and tooth caries. It resembles a fungus in its filamentous morphology but is related to the corynebacteria in the structure of its cell wall and its response to penicillin.

Chlamydial infection

These small obligate intracellular parasites have a curious lifestyle involving an initial infective elementary body, and a reticulate body which replicates to release more elementary bodies. *Chlamydia trachomatis*, primarily a genital infection, can spread to the eye to cause conjunctivitis and trachoma, the commonest cause of blindness—perhaps 5 000 000 cases worldwide. *C. psittaci* (acquired from birds) and *C. pneumoniae* are among the causes of atypical pneumonia.

Rickettsial infection

Rickettsiae are also obligate intracellular parasites because of a requirement for certain host cell factors (NAD, ATP, coenzyme A). They are acquired from animals or indirectly via insect bites. Brain, liver, and skin (vasculitis) are the organs chiefly affected. Different species cause slightly different diseases in different parts of the world (*Rickettsia rickettsii*: Rocky Mountain spotted fever; *R. conorii*: Mediterranean spotted fever; *R. typhi*, *R. prowazekii*: typhus; *R. tsutsugamushi*: scrub typhus; *Coxiella burnetii*: Q fever).

Mycoplasma

Mycoplasma are atypical in not possessing a normal bacterial cell wall. *M. pneumoniae* is an important cause of bronchitis and pneumonia. *M. hominis* may cause genital infections though this is disputed.

32 Fungal disease and immunity

Look back to Chapter 4 to be reminded that fungal diseases fall into three main patterns: *primary* infections in healthy individuals, viz: (1) filamentous moulds infecting the superficial and subcutaneous tissues, and (2) a dimorphic group causing systemic, mainly lung, infections; and (3) *secondary* infections caused by a number of important opportunists which have come to the fore with the increase in immunocompromised patients, in which they can cause disseminated and even fatal disease (Table 32.1). The mechanisms of host defence are generally similar to those that act against bacteria, namely the intact skin and membranes; antibody, complement, neutrophils, and macrophages for extracellular organisms; and T_H1 cells and cytokines for those that survive in macrophages. Escape mechanisms/virulence factors include immunosuppression (e.g. of T cells by dermatophytes), the production of capsules (by *Cryptococcus*), and inhibition of intracellular killing (e.g. by *Histoplasma*). In general, T_H1-type immunity correlates with effective immunity and T_H2-type with susceptibility; antibodies have been shown to be protective only in some cases, e.g. *Cryptococcus*.

Primary superficial and subcutaneous infections

Tinea (ringworm) is commoner in children than adults, partly because of the anti-fungal effect of post-pubertal sebaceous secretions. The occurrence of disseminated infection with *Trichophyton* spp. in immunocompromised patients suggests a role for immunity in normal individuals, but the precise mechanisms are unknown. Similarly, the mycetoma of *Madurella* and other species of mould (Madura foot) and the nodular lesions of *Sporothrix* (sporotrichosis), despite their granulomatous pathology, are commoner in patients with impaired cell-mediated immunity. *Candida albicans* is a rather special case, being a normal commensal of skin and mucous membranes, which can exacerbate to cause the itching and discharging lesions of *thrush*, frequently under the influence of antibiotic treatment, which suppresses the normal bacterial flora. However, systemic dissemination is seen in the immunocompromised, I/V drug users, and patients with cerebral lines.

Table 32.1 Some conditions predisposing to fungal infection

Condition	Common infections

T cell defects
  AIDS,
  Immunosuppressive drugs
	Aspergillus, Candida, Cryptococcus,
	Pneumocystis, Penicillium

Neutrophil defects	*Aspergillus; Candida; Zygomyces*
Diabetes	*Candida; Zygomyces*
Tumours	*Candida; Aspergillus*
Cystic fibrosis	*Aspergillus*
Antibacterial drug therapy	*Candida*
Surgery; catheters	*Candida*

Systemic infections

The dimorphic fungi *Histoplasma*, *Blastomyces*, and *Coccidioides*, mainly restricted to the American continent, exist in a filamentous form in soil, from which the spores, inhaled into the lung, develop into the yeast phase, giving rise to a pneumonia-like illness from which recovery is usual. A similar disease occurs following inhalation of the yeast *Cryptococcus*. Further dissemination, especially in the immunocompromised, may be fatal (see below). Thus, once again, there is good evidence for protective immunity. The increased susceptibility of AIDS patients, plus experiments in animal models, suggest a major role for CD4 T cells, mainly through their effect in activating the intracellular killing mechanisms in macrophages and neutrophils. *Histoplasma* is particularly prone to remain dormant for years after apparent recovery, and to flare up if immunodeficiency occurs.

Opportunistic infections

Here the evidence for protective immunity is strongest, since the fungi do not cause disease except in the immunocompromised.

Candidiasis

This is the predominant opportunistic fungal infection, particularly in hospitalized patients. It is common in T cell deficiencies, particularly AIDS, but also in patients on steroids or antibiotics, drug abusers, diabetics, leukaemics, and post-operatively. The lesions may affect the skin and mucous membranes (chronic mucocutaneous candidiasis; CMC) or the gastro-intestinal tract or, in severe cases, dissemination can occur to any organ, including the eye and heart.

Cryptococcus

Unlike most fungi, C. *neoformans* is susceptible to antibody and complement, since IgG against the polysaccharide capsule can overcome its anti-phagocytic effect. However, T_H1 cells and cytokines are also involved in its control, and spread outside the lung, particularly to the meninges and brain, is common in AIDS patients.

Pneumocystis carinii

This organism, once considered a protozoan, has the dubious distinction of having led to the discovery of AIDS (see Chapter 25). In small numbers it is probably a normal resident of the lung in most individuals, but multiplies to cause severe pneumonia in T-cell deficient patients. There is debate as to whether this constitutes a reactivation of pre-existent organisms or a true reinfection.

Aspergillus

This filamentous mould can cause symptoms in four situations: (1) normal people may become allergic to the spores, mainly of A. *fumigatus*, and develop asthma; (2) in patients with pre-existing lung infection (e.g. cavitating TB) the hyphae may grow into a large *fungus ball*, worsening the respiratory problems; (3) in immunocompromised, particularly neutropaenic, individuals primary infection is often in the lungs and dissemination can occur to brain, heart, gut, and bone, with frequently fatal results; (4) the exotoxin (aflatoxin) of A. *flavus*, a contaminant of stored grain or nuts, is a risk factor for liver cancer.

Zygomycosis

A variety of filamentous fungi that are prone to infect and proliferate in injured, burned, malnourished, diabetic, and other debilitated patients, though less often in those with AIDS. Reduced neutrophil and macrophage function appears to be the common predisposing factor.

Treatment and vaccines

Anti-fungal chemotherapy is aimed predominantly at cell wall synthesis, but there are a few drugs that act against protein and nucleic acid synthesis; for further details see Chapter 28. There are no vaccines in use at present, but in experimental vaccine models both antibody-mediated (e.g. for *Cryptococcus*, *Candida*, *Aspergillus*) and cell-mediated immunity (e.g. for *Histoplasma*, *Blastomyces*, *Coccidioides*) have been induced. Another possibility is the use of monoclonal antibodies for passive immunization.

33 Protozoal disease and immunity

The common features of the protozoal pathogens described in Chapter 5 are that (1) the diseases they cause are extremely chronic, with spontaneous recovery a very rare event and only partial immunity at best, and (2) no effective vaccines are currently available. The problem lies in their highly developed *immune evasion* mechanisms, which make use of virtually all the devices discussed in Chapters 12 and 21.

Malaria

In populations regularly exposed to malaria, most deaths and severe complications (e.g. anaemia, cerebral malaria) and the highest parasitaemias are seen in children, suggesting that older patients have acquired some degree of immunity to both the parasite and the disease. This immunity is maintained by continued exposure to infection and can be lost after only a few months of non-exposure. Experiments in mice suggest that T cells, antibody, and cytokines all play a role (Fig. 33.1). The continued survival of parasites in patients with high levels of antibody and activated T cells is due to a number of factors:

1. Following a mosquito bite, the survival of only a few sporozoites is enough to initiate a liver-stage infection.
2. The free-living blood stages (sporozoite, merozoite) are very brief—seconds or minutes.
3. The intracellular liver stage is susceptible to killing by CD8 T cells and activated macrophages, but only a few released merozoites are needed to initiate the blood-stage infection.
4. Both the free merozoite and the infected red cells carry dominant antigens which are highly polymorphic and may undergo variation. Polymorphism is enhanced by the presence of a sexual stage in the cycle.
5. Malaria infection is immunosuppressive.

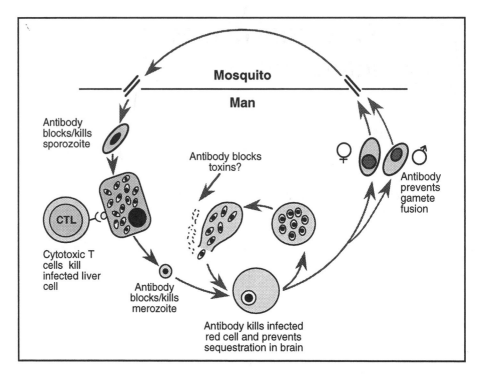

Fig. 33.1 The malaria life cycle offers numerous points of attack for the immune system.

Prospects for a vaccine

A vaccine that prevented malaria, or prevented the million or more deaths per year from malaria, or even reduced transmission, would be of enormous benefit. There is no shortage of potential parasite antigens, as Table 33.1 shows, but trials to date have been disappointing. Current hopes are pinned on combinations of three or more antigens plus novel delivery systems.

Immunopathology

Apart from the anaemia, which is partly due to direct destruction of red cells, the symptoms and complications of malaria are related to immune activity, particularly (1) immune complex formation, leading to glomerulonephritis, and (2) excessive release of inflammatory cytokines such as TNFα, IL-1, IL-6, and IFNγ, which underlie the fever, the hypoglycaemia, and probably the cerebral changes. Unfortunately, several anti-TNF antibody trials in humans have only reduced fever and not mortality. The reason for the chronic nephrotic syndrome caused by *P. malariae* is not understood. The link between malaria, EB virus, and Burkitt's lymphoma is thought to be at least partly due to suppression of the CTL

Table 33.1 Potential target antigens for malarial immunity and vaccination

Source	Antigen	Role of immunity if successful
Sporozoite	CSP; TRAP	Antibody blocks entry into liver cell
Liver cell	LSA-1	CD8+ T cells kill infected liver cell
Merozoite	MSP-1;2;4	Antibody blocks entry into red cell
	EBA-175	" " " " " "
	AMA-1	" " " " " "
Infected red cell	PfEMP-1	Antibody blocks sequestration
Gametocyte	Pfs 230; 48/45	Prevents sexual stage and transmission
Gamete	Pfg 25/27	" " " " "

response to EBV-infected B lymphocytes. Early in the twentieth century, controlled *P. vivax* infection ('fever therapy') was used to treat late-stage syphilis, on the basis that treponemes survive poorly at high temperatures.

Treatment

Both the liver and the blood stage are susceptible to drugs, but resistance has developed to most of these (see Chapter 28).

Leishmaniasis

The critical element in leishmaniasis is survival of the amastigote stage of the parasite within macrophages, which can be overcome by vigorous activation of the macrophages by cytokines, particularly IFNγ and TNF; hence the importance of T cells of the T_H1 subset. By contrast, T_H2 cells, by releasing IL-4, tend to promote non-protective antibody formation. In line with this, recovery and resistance correlate with strong delayed hypersensitivity responses. Encouragingly, only about 5% of exposed individuals develop disease. In immunodeficient patients (e.g. AIDS) both cutaneous and visceral disease are much more severe. The search for a vaccine has been encouraged by the fact that mild cases of *L. tropica* ('oriental sore') are immune to reinfection after recovery; deliberate exposure has traditionally been practised in the Middle East—a process known as 'leishmanization', analogous to the use of vaccinia against smallpox. There have been numerous trials of more sophisticated vaccines, but none has yet been adopted as standard. In their absence, treatment relies on antimonial drugs and the more expensive amphotericin B.

African trypanosomiasis

The two species of *T. brucei* are unique among protozoa in living and multiplying free in the blood, where they are exposed to virtually every element of the immune system, including antibody, complement, PMN, and lymphocytes. Their survival is due to a remarkable form of antigenic variation in which the parasite repeatedly changes its entire surface coat of 'variant specific glycoprotein' (VSG) by a gene switching mechanism; the genome contains about 1000 different genes for this purpose. As a result, following an antibody response, many parasites are eliminated but a new variant population emerges. The host is thus obliged to mount a series of primary responses at approximately weekly intervals (see Fig. 21.3). Massive polyclonal IgM production adds further to the inefficiency of immunity, the parasite stimulates inflammatory changes in the CNS, and the patient eventually succumbs to the coma of *sleeping sickness*. The prospects for a vaccine seem rather remote, and treatment is mainly based on arsenical drugs.

South American trypanosomiasis (Chagas' disease)

In its early stage in macrophages, *T. cruzi* behaves like *Leishmania*, inhibiting both intracellular killing mechanisms and their stimulation by IFNγ. The succeeding blood stage is resistant to lysis by complement, and the final stages in heart and nervous tissue are thought by some to cause their chronic destructive effects (cardiomegaly, megacolon), which may progress for decades, via *cross-reaction* between parasite and host antigens, leading to *autoimmunity*. Clearly a vaccine which enhanced this would be disastrous, and though arsenicals and other drugs are of some benefit, ultimate control of the disease lies in the hands of those responsible for the slum housing in which the reduviid bug vector flourishes.

Toxoplasmosis

Toxoplasma is of special interest as an intracellular parasite, able to develop in many types of cell and many species of animal. It is also an *opportunist*, taking advantage of weakened immunity to reactivate and proliferate, particularly in the brain (encephalitis) and eye (chorioretinitis). Toxoplasma is one of the few pathogens able to cross the placenta, infect the fetus, and cause malformations or neonatal infection—others being rubella virus, CMV, HIV, hepatitis B, syphilis, leprosy, and *Listeria*. Various drugs are used for treatment and prophylaxis, notably pyrimethamine–sulphonamide combinations such as co-trimoxazole. Care in handling pet cats, the definitive hosts and frequently carriers, is important for susceptible individuals.

Amoebiasis and giardiasis

Infection with *Entamoeba histolytica* can range from symptomless carriage, mild attacks of diarrhoea, and dysentery with bleeding, to peritonitis and abscesses in liver, lung, etc., with little evidence of useful immunity. Treatment with antibiotics and normal hygienic measures are the mainstay of control. *G. lamblia* causes a brief attack of diarrhoea, except in some immunodeficient patients when it may be prolonged and debilitating.

Cryptosporidiosis

Infection with *C. parvum*, which normally induces a brief episode of profuse diarrhoea, has emerged as an important cause of disease in AIDS patients, with additional dissemination to liver and lungs. Anti-HIV drugs give the best hope of recovery.

34 Helminth disease and immunity

As emphasized in Chapter 6, these large multicellular parasites represent a formidable challenge to the immune system, and such effective immunity as can be demonstrated is usually directed against the more delicate larval stages. Though differing in detail, worm infections have several features in common: (1) well-developed *evasion* mechanisms leading to chronicity; (2) a bias towards the T_H2 type of adaptive response, featuring the cytokines IL-3, 4, 5, 9 and 13, elevated numbers of mast cells and eosinophils, and high levels of IgE; (3) a tendency to induce strong *immunopathology*; and (4) a varying degree of *immunosuppression*.

Schistosomiasis

Estimates of the adult worm burden, derived from counting eggs in the faeces, show that in endemic areas the burden peaks in the mid-teens and then declines. This used to be attributed to differences in contact with the lake water in which the snail vector releases the infective cercaria (see Fig. 6.1 for the life cycle), plus a possible effect of pubertal sex hormones, but careful epidemiological studies suggest that there is also an element of true immunological resistance. This appears to act against the larval stage (schistosomulum), involving (1) killing in the skin by combinations such as specific IgE–eosinophils–major basic protein, specific IgG–macrophages–nitric oxide, and (2) interference with migration of the larvae through the lungs by inflammatory reactions. Younger stages are more susceptible than older ones, so that established worms survive in the presence of immunity against subsequent infections, a situation known as *concomitant immunity*. This survival by organisms lying within blood vessels is aided by the acquisition of host molecules, including blood group and MHC antigens, fibronectin, cholesterol, and non-specific immunoglobulins; thus the worm becomes 'camouflaged' by what to the host is 'self' material.

Immunopathology

Schistosomiasis would not be such a serious disease but for the fact that some eggs, instead of penetrating host tissues to reach the exterior, become trapped in organs such as the gut wall, liver (*S. mansoni*, *S. japonicum*), and bladder (*S. haematobium*). Here they provoke granuloma formation, again predominantly involving T_H2 cells, and cytokines (IL-4,5,13) and eosinophils. In the bladder this can lead to haematuria, urinary obstruction, calcification and, particularly in North Africa, bladder cancer. In the liver the granulomata may coalesce around the portal tracts to produce the classic 'pipe-stem fibrosis', leading to portal hypertension, dilated oesophageal varices, and haematemesis. There is some evidence that T_H1 cytokines (e.g. IFNγ) can slow the process of granuloma formation, but with this comes the danger of liver damage by molecules released by the eggs, since one of the effects of the granuloma is to wall off these toxic factors (Fig. 34.1).

Control and prospects for a vaccine

The evidence for at least partial immunity during natural infections is encouraging, and in animal models infection with X-irradiated cercariae, which mature to

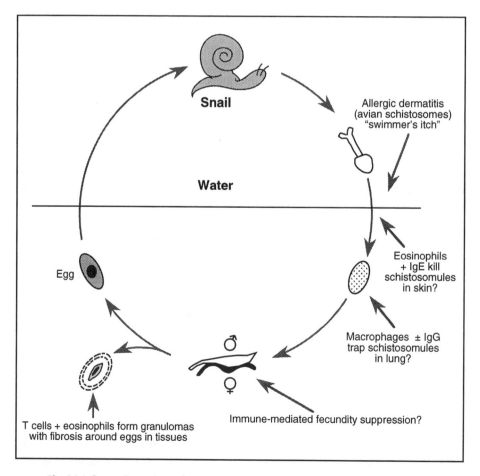

Fig. 34.1 Immunity against schistosomiasis can be both protective and pathological.

the lung stage and then die, induces up to 90% protection against subsequent challenge. Human studies have concentrated on purified or recombinant vaccine candidate antigens, notably the enzyme glutathione-S-transferase and the muscle protein paramyosin. An alternative idea, still experimental, is to try and reduce immunopathology by boosting T_H1 responses—an 'anti-disease' vaccine which might reduce the amount of fibrosis around trapped eggs. Fortunately there are safe and effective drugs, notably praziquantel, which kill adult worms. Public health measures to prevent contact between man and cercariae would constitute the ideal control strategy.

Filariasis

More is known about pathological than protective immunity against filarial nematodes, but encouragingly only a small proportion of exposed individuals actually develop symptoms, suggesting that immunopathological responses are under the influence of genetic and/or environmental factors.

Lymphatic filariasis

Simple blockage of lymphatics by adult *Wuchereria* worms is not enough to explain the swelling and hardening of tissues seen in elephantiasis, and there is probably an element of chronic inflammation due to superimposed bacterial and fungal infection. The presence in the soil of quartz, which is toxic to macrophages, is thought to be another factor. However, elephantiasis is rare, and many exposed individuals clear their worms, retaining high levels of specific IgE and T_H2 cytokine responses. Others have circulating microfilariae and only minor lymphatic pathology, with suppressed T_H1 responses (e.g. IFNγ), not only to worm antigens but unrelated antigens such as BCG; this is associated with high levels of IL-10. Interestingly, most filarial worms carry the endosymbiotic rickettsia *Wolbachia*, which produces an LPS that may contribute to inflammation. A few patients with extremely high levels of IgE and eosinophils develop a severe allergic response to microfilariae in the lung known as tropical pulmonary eosinophilia.

Onchocerciasis

The most serious complication is *river blindness*, so named because the fly vector breeds in running water and the microfilariae migrate to the skin and eye, where they provoke damage which may be partly immunological—Types I, III, and IV hypersensitivity have all been postulated. In endemic areas 2–5% of children and 4–14% of adults are blind—an incidence three times higher than for trachoma. Treatment with diethylcarbamizide, which kills microfilariae, used to be followed by an acute reaction in the skin (Mazzotti reaction) apparently due to allergy to released worm antigens.

Current therapy for filariasis favours the drug ivermectin and programmes have been proposed for its free distribution.

Intestinal nematode infections

Evidence for a role of immunity in human nematode infections comes from the effect of *immunodeficiency* on strongyloidiasis, which became apparent with the introduction of steroid treatment in the 1960s, resulting in massive body-wide fatal larval burdens. Whether this is due to reduced larval killing (e.g. by IgE) or increased worm fecundity is not clear. A similar effect is not seen with *Ascaris*, *Trichuris*, etc., but about 10% of normal individuals have unusually high worm counts, possibly for genetic or immunological reasons. In animal models, a number of factors contribute to the killing and expulsion of worms, including the activity of T_H2 cells in increasing IgE, mucin production, smooth muscle contraction, and lipid peroxidation of the worm membrane. There is some evidence that IgE can reduce the egg output of female hookworms. Passage of *Ascaris* through the lungs can trigger pulmonary eosinophilia with asthma (Loeffler's syndrome). Drug-treatment of *Ascaris* has been shown to improve the response to a cholera vaccine and to BCG, suggesting that here, too, the suppression of T_H1 responsiveness, e.g. by IL-10, is of general significance.

Hydatid disease

The hydatid cysts of *Echinococcus granulosus* (see Chapter 6) may rupture, particularly during surgical removal, releasing worm antigens into the circulation. Because of the already-present high levels of specific IgE on mast cells, massive life-threatening anaphylaxis may follow (see Fig. 22.2). It has been shown that injection of serum from a patient into his own cyst can result in killing of the worms in it; thus the cyst constitutes a protected site for the worms in an otherwise hostile environment. An experimental vaccine is under development for use in dogs.

Worms and allergy

It has frequently been observed that allergies are less common in the tropics, but the earlier hypothesis that the high levels of circulating IgE blocked receptors on mast cells has not been upheld; alternative proposals are (1) raised levels of IL-10, and (2) direct effects of worm products on eosinophils.

35 Emerging and future infectious diseases

The delicate balance between infectious organisms and human populations, as we have described it in this book, has been gradually established over hundreds of thousands of years. However, it is still possible for the infectious disease profile of a population to undergo sudden alterations for a number of reasons:

(1) The causative organism may be identified for a previously unrecognized disease;

(2) A pathogen previously restricted to animals (zoonosis) may cross into humans;

(3) New opportunistic infections may appear in immunocompromised patients;

(4) A known organism may increase its virulence by mutation or gene transfer;

(5) A new organism may be created accidentally or deliberately;

(6) An organism may change its resistance to chemotherapy;

(7) A vaccine campaign may be abandoned;

(8) Public health measures may break down;

(9) Travel brings host and pathogen together for the first time;

(10) Climatic changes; global warming.

In this chapter we will consider the major changes that have occurred within living memory—always bearing in mind that *all* infections make their first appearance in a population at *some* date. For example in 1347 the arrival of plague from the East must have been even more unexpected and terrifying to Europeans than the arrival of HIV to us. However, plague is rather exceptional and probably most of today's human diseases go back to prehistoric times; polio, schistosomiasis and tuberculosis can be clearly recognized in ancient Egyptian documents. Domestication of animals and the setting up of closely packed urban communities around 10 000 years ago were probably the major factors in establishing the present pattern of human infections.

Newly identified pathogens

Several microorganisms have only been identified as the cause of disease in recent years; Tables 35.1 and 35.2 list the most important of these.

Table 35.1 Some recently identified human pathogens

Organism	Disease
Borrelia burgdorferi (1975)	Lyme disease
Legionella pneumophila (1976)	Legionnaire's disease
Helicobacter pylori (1983)	Gastric ulcer and cancer
Hepatitis C (1989); D,E	Hepatitis
HHV 6 (1988); 7	Roseola infantum
HHV 8 (1995)	Kaposi's sarcoma
SARS coronavirus (2003)	SARS

Newly acquired zoonoses

Unusual contacts with animals—e.g. African monkeys shipped to laboratories in Europe—have caused sporadic cases of severe disease, often haemorrhagic and fatal (Table 35.2). The proposed use of animal organs for transplantation, and in particular those of pigs, which have been genetically modified to be more suitable

Table 35.2 Some recently identified zoonotic infections

Organism	Source	Disease
West Nile virus (1937)	Birds	Encephalitis
Marburg virus (1967)	African green monkeys	Haemorrhagic fever
Lassa fever virus (1969)	Rodents	Haemorrhagic fever; shock
Monkeypox (1970)	Monkeys, squirrels	Like smallpox
Ebola virus (1976)	?Bats; monkeys	Haemorrhagic fever
Hanta virus (1978)	Rodents	Pulmonary syndrome
HIV 1, 2 (1981)	Chimpanzees, monkeys	AIDS
Hendra virus (1994)	Horses	Respiratory
Variant CJD (1995)	Cattle	Spongiform encephalitis
Nipah virus (1998)	Pigs	Encephalitis

donors, is a potential source of new virus infections, though no evidence for this has yet emerged.

Opportunistic infections

During the last 50 years the number of immunocompromised individuals in the population has increased tremendously, for three reasons: (1) improved diagnosis, treatment, and survival of primary immunodeficiencies; (2) the widespread use of immunosuppressive drugs for transplantation, cancer therapy, and inflammatory disease; (3) the AIDS epidemic. In such patients, in addition to unusually severe infections with normal pathogens, a variety of organisms previously considered harmless can become pathogenic (Table 35.3).

Table 35.3 Some important opportunistic infections (see also Table 25.7)

Organism	Disease in immunocompromised host
Cytomegalovirus (HHV 5)	Pneumonitis; fetal abnormalities
HSV	Generalized herpes
VZV	Generalized VZV; shingles
EBV	Burkitt's lymphoma
Mycobacterium avium-intracellulare	disseminated infection
Pseudomonas aeruginosa	Skin infection; pneumonia; septicaemia
Proteus	Pneumonia
Candida albicans	Chronic mucocutaneous candidiasis
Cryptococcus neoformans	Pneumonia; meningitis
Pneumocystis carinii	Pneumonia
Cryptosporidium	Diarrhoea
Giardia lamblia	Diarrhoea
Toxoplasma gondii	Brain, eye defects, also in fetus
Strongyloides	Diarrhoea, malabsorption, dissemination

Changes in virulence

Here the classic example is influenza, where each pandemic is due to what is essentially a new recombinant virus ('antigenic shift', see Chapter 21)—some, such as the 'Spanish' H1N1 strain of 1918, the 'Asian' H2N2 of 1957, and the 'Hong Kong' H3N2 of 1968 being particularly virulent. The latter two strains were recombinants between avian and human viruses, but the 1918 strain, which killed 5% of the world population, is believed to have been an unaltered porcine virus and should therefore be considered as a zoonosis. At the time of writing (2003) a new coronavirus, originating in China, is causing a pandemic of *severe acute respiratory syndrome* (SARS) with a mortality of around 4%. This is worrying because coronaviruses, a common cause of colds, are not normally fatal. One possibility is that, as with flu, an animal or bird virus is involved. If so, this is a further warning that close human–animal contact is a potent source of danger.

Artificial creation of new pathogen

Every attenuated vaccine is in effect a new organism, deliberately created to be immunogenic but not virulent. However, when inadvertently given to immuno-compromised individuals, it can give rise to a new disease (e.g. disseminated BCG-osis in T-cell deficient babies). With the development of recombinant DNA technology it has become possible to create new organisms of increased virulence for use in biological warfare, for instance by incorporating genes for immune or antibiotic resistance. Increased virulence can also be introduced accidentally; for example a vaccinia virus incorporating the gene for IL-4, which was expected to improve its antigenicity, was actually *more* lethal in mice—in effect a new 'killer virus'. In addition a number of naturally occurring pathogens are under consideration as biological weapons of mass destruction (Table 35.4).

Table 35.4 Some candidate agents for biological warfare

Pathogen/disease	Type of agent	Comments
Anthrax	Bacterium	Easily spread; high mortality
Plague	Bacterium	″ ″ ″ ″
Tularemia	Bacterium	Easily spread; low mortality
Botulism	Bacterial toxin	High mortality
Smallpox	Virus	Easily spread but vaccine available
Haemorrhagic fevers	Virus	Easily spread; no available treatment
Burkholderia		
mallei	Bacteria	Easily spread; often fatal
pseudomallei	Bacteria	″ ″ ″ ″
Ricin	Plant toxin	More suitable for use on individuals

Drug resistance

The widespread use of antibiotics has had an enormous effect on the world of pathogens, promoting the emergence of resistant strains that may eventually replace the original population. Multiple-drug-resistant staphylococci and tubercle bacilli are leading examples (see Chapter 28). If the drug-resistant strain also happens to have a growth advantage in normal hosts, it would spread through untreated populations very rapidly; this may have been the case with chloroquine resistance in malaria.

Vaccine uptake

The reduction in disease following a successful vaccine campaign can easily be reversed if for some reason vaccine uptake is reduced. This is usually either because the disease is no longer seen as a threat (e.g. diphtheria in developed countries) or because the vaccine is considered, rightly or wrongly, to be dangerous. Examples of this are the pertussis 'scare' of 1978 (see Chapter 27) and the recent claim of a link between the MMR vaccine, bowel disease, and autism which, though not upheld by further studies, has prejudiced some parents against the measles component of the vaccine, and has led to an increase in cases of the disease.

Public health

Public health measures require considerable political will for their maintenance. Food and water hygiene and vector control can easily break down in the face of other priorities such as war or revolution. Even in peacetime, education of the public about the cause and transmission of disease is not always the priority it should be—and here newspapers do not help by publishing inaccurate stories and spreading unjustified 'scares'. On the other hand, delay by health authorities or governments in admitting that outbreaks have occurred, usually because of embarrassment, can seriously endanger attempts at proper control. Recent examples are BSE in the UK, SARS in China and AIDS in S. Africa.

Travel and immigration

Most infectious diseases have a sufficiently long incubation for a tourist or immigrant to start his or her journey healthy and become ill after arrival. There have been cases where tourists spent a single night in a tropical hotel and died of malaria, sometimes undiagnosed and not even suspected, in their home town. In the absence of breeding mosquitoes, this would not pose a danger to the public, but many pathogens can maintain themselves in a new habitat, for example the West Nile encephalitis virus in humans and animals, recently imported for the first time (1999) into the USA and now successfully established there.

Climate

One of the perils of global warming will probably be the appearance of 'tropical' diseases in temperate countries whose inhabitants, genetically and immunologically unprepared for the new pathogens, would be expected to suffer worse disease than those in the tropical areas that have had thousands of years to adapt. Possibly immigrant populations from these endemic areas would find themselves at an advantage.

Without wishing to appear unduly fatalistic, we hope we have made clear in this chapter that the host–pathogen balance is never in a stationary state. The tireless efforts of generations of microbiologists, epidemiologists, immunologists, and health workers of all kinds have achieved reductions in infectious disease undreamed of in earlier times, but there is plenty of opportunity for the trend to be reversed if vigilance is not maintained.

Tutorial 4

This section of the book has a more 'clinical' feel which may disconcert those with no medical knowledge. By attempting the following essays, you may find you know more than you thought about the clinical implications of infection. In any case there is no harm in knowing about medical and health matters, provided you remember to let your doctor feel he knows more than you do (which he probably does).

1. 'Money should go into public health measures rather than drugs or vaccines.' Should it?
2. '. . . the death of the child appearing to be inevitable . . . on July 6 . . . little Meister was inoculated ... with a half-full syringe of spinal cord from a rabbit dead of rabies . . . preserved in a dry air flask . . . Joseph Meister escaped the rabies . . .' (Pasteur 1885). Explain this happy outcome.
3. 'The golden age of antibiotics is past.' Is it?
4. 'Eucaryotic infections are the worst.' Are they?
5. 'AIDS is the most serious infectious disease we have ever encountered.' Do you agree?
6. What further improvements in the immune system might evolve, given time?

Some guides to a possible answer.

1. In a Utopia where everyone has unlimited access to clean water and properly cooked food, every wound is promptly sterilized, and everyone with the slightest infection is rigorously isolated until they either recover or die, we probably could manage quite well without vaccines or antibiotics. However, it is hard to imagine such conditions ever being established, let alone maintained. There is certainly an argument for *fewer* drugs and perhaps fewer vaccines, and there is a strong argument for much more information on, and enforcement of public health measures. A safe guide might be that the latter should replace the former *when possible*.
2. Pasteur was amazingly lucky! His dried rabbit spinal cord contained dead rabies virus—a very hazardous way of killing an organism nobody at that time had ever seen. He was using it as a vaccine in a child already exposed by the bite of a rabid dog. In any other infection this would be too late for active

immunization, but rabies has an unusually long incubation period, giving the immune system time to respond before symptoms appear. Killed virus is still used to protect against rabies, combined with passive antibody if exposure has already occurred.

3. This frequently heard statement reflects the fact that resistance eventually develops to virtually all antibiotics, especially when they are used carelessly. It is somewhat over-defeatist, in that millions of lives are still saved every year by the correct use of antibiotics, and the pharmaceutical industry is continually producing new antibiotics, based on ever-improving knowledge of microbial biology. If there ever was a golden age, it was founded more on ignorance and optimism than on fact. In any case, where eucaryotic organisms are concerned, the golden age has hardly begun.

4. It depends what you mean by *worst*. The top killers at present (HIV, TB, infantile diarrhoea) are viruses or bacteria, i.e. *not* eucaryotes—although the top eucaryote (malaria) runs them close. The thought behind this statement was probably that eucaryotic infections (fungal, protozoal, helminth) are the hardest to *treat*, either with drugs or vaccines, whereas there is a steadily increasing list of effective drugs and/or vaccines against viruses and bacteria. Another problem is that because of their means of transmission, protozoal and helminth infections tend to be commonest in tropical countries, where adequate funding for health care is not always available.

5. One is certainly tempted to agree with this statement. What is so alarming about HIV is that, as a newcomer to the human race and already the leading single infectious cause of death, what it will do next is still unknown. Really vigorous public health measures and the provision of cheap effective drugs will undoubtedly slow its progress, and reduction of secondary infections will prolong lives (in fact the really devastating threat is the combination of HIV and tuberculosis). An effective vaccine would change everything though the prospects are not too good (why is this?). In the *very* long term there will probably be selection for resistance genes. You could argue that plague in the Middle Ages and influenza in 1918 were almost as bad, and if they had been sexually transmitted they might have been. But if one wished to invent a truly ruthless and terrifying pathogen, it would be hard to improve on HIV.

6. A fascinating challenge, tempting the unwary to invent all kinds of exotic new cells and molecules. However, you will find that most 'improvements' bring with them new risks in the shape of immunopathology, autoimmunity, etc. In the process, you will come to appreciate just how well-designed the immune system is. The safest bet is probably a continuation of existing trends such as (1) more V genes in the germ line (a rare event, requiring a useful mutation during gametogenesis), (2) another immunoglobulin C gene, conferring some new biological property on the antibody molecule—different species of mammals already differ considerably in their IgG subclass genes, showing that they are fairly recent developments, (3) some more natural inhibitors of en-

dotoxin and other life-threatening molecules, (4) further diversification of the MHC (which would benefit the species rather than the individual). In the very long term, it would be nice to imagine some way in which the brain could acquire more control over the immune system.

Looking at it from the therapeutic viewpoint, we might expect to see (1) a reliable way of directing vaccines at T_H1, T_H2, and B cells, (2) a safe way of switching on and enhancing NK cell activity, (3) safe, efficient gene replacement for the congenital immunodeficiencies, (4) a range of monoclonal antibodies against infectious organisms—though admittedly the existing monoclonals have not been as successful as was hoped.

Appendix 1
The major causes of human infection

Upper respiratory tract

Rhinovirus
Coronavirus
Adenovirus
Echovirus
Coxsackie virus
EB virus
Influenza virus
Strep. pyogenes
Haemophilus influenzae
Diphtheria

Lower respiratory tract

Influenza; parainfluenza
Respiratory syncytial
    virus (RSV)
Measles virus
Adenovirus; rhinovirus
Strep. pneumoniae
Bordetella pertussis
Haemophilus
Staph. aureus
M. tuberculosis
Legionella
Pseudomonas

Ear infection

Mumps virus
RSV
Strep. pneumoniae

Eye infection

Adenovirus
Measles virus
Strep. pneumoniae
Trachoma
Toxoplasma
Onchocerca

Meningitis & encephalitis

Herpesvirus
Varicella-zoster virus
Measles virus
HIV
Polio virus
Rabies virus
M. tuberculosis
N. meningitidis
Haemophilus
Malaria
Trypanosomiasis
Toxoplasma

Gastroenteritis

Rotavirus
Salmonella spp.
Shigella
E. coli
V. cholerae
Campylobacter
Helicobacter
Entamoeba
Giardia
Cryptosporidium
Strongyloides

Food poisoning

Staph. aureus
B. cereus
C. botulinum

Urinary infection

E. coli
Proteus
Staphylococci

Sexually transmitted

Herpesvirus 1, 2
HIV
Hepatitis B
Genital warts
N. gonorrhoeae
Syphilis
Chlamydia
Candida
Trichomonas

Appendix 2
Cytokines featured in this book
(see also Tables 11.2, 18.1, 19.1)

Cytokine	Main cell source	Main functions
IL 1	Mac	Acute phase response, fever
IL 2	T	B cell activation; T and NK cell proliferation
IL 3	T	Haemopoiesis
IL 4	TH2, NKT	TH2 differentiation; B cell activation, Ig switch
IL 5	TH2	B cell, eosinophil growth; IgA switch
IL 6	T, Mac	B cell, plasma cell differentiation; acute phase response
IL 7	Bone marrow	Early T, B cell maturation
IL 8	Leukocytes	Cell migration
IL 10	TH2	B cell proliferation
		Macrophage inhibition
IL 12	Mac, DC,	TH1, NK activation
IL 13	TH2	IgE switch; macrophage inhibition
IL 15	Mac	T, NK proliferation
IL 17	Memory T	Induction of IL1, TNF, chemokines
IL 18	Mac, DC	T, NK activation
IL 23	Mac, DC	TH1, memory T differentiation
IFNα	Mac	Anti-viral, TH1
IFNβ	Fibroblasts	Anti-viral
IFNγ	TH1, NK, CTL	Anti-viral, B cell IgG switch
		Macrophage activation
TNF	T, DC	Acute phase response, inflammation
TGFβ	T, Mac	B cell IgA switch
		Inhibit T, macrophages

IL: interleukin; IFN: interferon; TNF: tumour necrosis factor; TGF: transforming growth factor; Mac: macrophage; DC: dendritic cell; NK: natural killer cell

Appendix 3
Cluster of differentiation (CD) antigens.
Over 250 of these have been identified. The following are those mentioned in this book

CD number	Other names	Cell distribution	Main functions/ comments
1		T, B, DC	Presentation of glyco lipid antigens
2	LFA2	T, NK	Costimulation
3		T,	Linked to T cell receptor
4		T helper	Binds to MHC II; also receptor for HIV
8		Cytotoxic T	Binds to MHC I
14		DC, mono, mac, gran	LPS binding
16	FcγRIII	NK, Mac	Aids phagocytosis
19		B	Costimulation of B cells
21	CR2	B	Aids antigen uptake
23	Fcε receptor	B, Mac	low affinity IgE receptor
28		T, B	Costimulation
32	Fcγ RIIr	Mac, B, Eos	Aids phagocytosis
35	CR 1	Mac, B	Aids phagocytosis
44		Memory T	leucocyte adhesion
45		Leucocytes	lymphocyte activation
46		Widespread	Regulates complement; also receptor for measles virus
64	FcγRI	Mac	Aids phagocytosis
81		T, B	Costimulation
89	FcRα	Mac,	Cytotoxicity

DC: dendritic cell; NK: natural killer cell; Eos: eosinophil; FcR: receptor for Ig Fc region; CR: receptor for complement; Gran: granulocyte

Further reading and information

Part I   The infectious organisms

Textbooks

- Brock Biology of Microorganisms. M. T. Madigan, J. M. Martinko, and J. Parker Pearson Education, 10th edn., 2003.
- Medical Microbiology. C. Mims, H. Dockrell, R. Gotting I. Roitt, D. Wakelin, and M. Zuckerman, Moseby 3rd ed., 2004.
- The Pathogenesis of Infectious Disease. C. A. Mims, A. Nash, and J. Stephen, Academic Press, 5th ed., 2001.

Web sites

- www.hhmi.org/lectures/1999/index.htm (Topics in microbial pathogenesis, with video clips).
- www.microbeworld.org/home.htm (general American Society for Microbiology sponsored site on current topics in microbiology. See also ASM home page at www.asm.org)
- www.sanger.ac.uk/ (The Wellcome Trust Sanger Institute. Sequencing of microbial genomes.)
- www.tigr.org/ (The Institute for Genomic Research (TIGR). Sequencing of microbial genomes.)

Recent Reviews and Articles

- Wren, B. W. 'Microbial genome analysis: insights into virulence, host adaptation and evolution'. *Nature Reviews Genetics*, 2000, 1:30.
- Blackwell, J. M. 'Genetics and genomics in infectious disease susceptibility'. *Trends Mol. Med.*, 2001, Nov. 7 (11): 521–6.
- Florens, L., Washburn, M. P., Raine, J. D., Anthony, R. M., Grainger, M., Haynes, J. D., Moch, J. K., Muster, N., Sacci, J. B., Tabb, D. L., Witney, A. A., Wolters, D., Wu, Y., Gardner, M. J., Holder, A. A., Sinden, R. E., Yates, J. R., Carucci, D. J. 'A proteomic view of the Plasmodium falciparum life cycle'. *Nature*. 2002, Oct. 3; 419 (6906): 520–6.
- Gardner, M. J., Hall, N., Fung, E., White, O., Berriman, M., Hyman, R. W., Carlton, J. M., Pain, A., Nelson, K. E., Bowman, S., Paulsen, I. T., James, K.,

Eisen, J. A., Rutherford, K., Salzberg, S. L., Craig, A., Kyes, S., Chan, M. S., Nene, V., Shallom, S. J., Suh, B., Peterson, J., Angiuoli, S., Pertea, M., Allen, J., Selengut, J., Haft, D., Mather, M. W., Vaidya, A. B., Martin, D. M., Fairlamb, A. H., Fraunholz, M. J., Roos, D. S., Ralph, S. A., McFadden, G. I., Cummings, L. M., Subramanian, G. M., Mungall, C., Venter, J. C., Carucci, D. J., Hoffman, S. L., Newbold, C., Davis, R. W., Fraser, C. M., Barrell, B. 'Genome sequence of the human malaria parasite Plasmodium falciparum'. *Nature*. 2002, Oct. 3; 419 (6906): 498–511.

- Cole, S. T. 'Comparative and functional genomics of the Mycobacterium tuberculosis complex'. *Microbiology*. 2002, Oct. 148 (Pt 10): 2919–28.

- Gauthier, A., Thomas, N. A., Finlay, B. B. 'Bacterial injection machines'. *J. Biol Chem*. 2003, May 19.

- Pannifer, A. D., Wong, T. Y., Schwarzenbacher, R., Renatus, M., Petosa, C., Bienkowska, J., Lacy, D. B., Collier, R. J., Park, S., Leppla, S. H., Hanna, P., Liddington, R. C. 'Crystal structure of the anthrax lethal factor'. *Nature*. 2001, Nov. 8; 414 (6860): 229–33.

Part 2   The immune system

Textbooks

- *Immunology*. Goldsby, R. A., Kindt, T. J., Osborne, B. A. and Kuby, J. W. H. Freeman. 5th edn., 2003.

- *Immunobiology: the immune system in health and disease*. Janeway, C. A., Travers, P., Walport, M., Shlomchik, M. Garland, 5th edn. 2001.

- *Immunology of Infectious Diseases*. Kaufmann, S. H. E., Sher, A. and Ahmed, R. ASM Press. 2002.

- *Cellular and Molecular Immunology*. Abbas A. K., Lichtman A. H. Saunders, 5th edn, 2003.

Websites

- http://image.bloodline.net/ (colour images of blood cell morphology.)

- www.cellsalive.com/clips.htm (commercial website offering video images of events in microbiology and immunology such as phagocyte chemotaxis, cytotoxic T cell killing, etc.)

- www.immunology.org/ (website of the British Society for Immunology.)

- http://12.17.12.70/aai (website of the American Association of Immunologists.)

- www.niaid.nih.gov/default.htm (website for the National Institute of Allergy and Infectious Diseases (National Institutes of Health, USA).)

- www.rndsystems.com/asp/g_sitebuilder.asp?BodyId=2 (R&D systems site offering succinct reviews with colour figures on cytokine biology and other topics in immunology and inflammation such as wound healing, etc.)

- http://research.bmn.com/mkmd (extensive list and details of knockout mice.)

Recent Reviews and Articles
Innate immunity

- Barton, G. M., Medzhitov, R. 'Toll-like receptors and their ligands'. *Curr. Top. Microbiol. Immunol.* 2002; 270: 81–92.

- Medzhitov, R., Janeway, C. A. Jr. 'Decoding the patterns of self and nonself by the innate immune system'. *Science.* 2002, Apr. 12; 296 (5566): 298–300.

- McCormack, F. X. and Whitsett, J. A. 'The pulmonary collectins, SP-A and SP-D orchestrate innate immunity in the lung'. *J. Clin. Invest.* 2002; 109: 707.

- Fujita, T. 'Evolution of the lectin-complement pathway and its role in innate immunity'. *Nature Reviews Immunol.* 2002; 2: 346.

- Chensue. 'Molecular machinations: Chemokine signals in Host-Pathogen interactions'. *Clinical Microbiology Reviews* 2001; 14(4) :821.

- Colucci, F., Di Santo, J. P., and Leibson, P. J. 'Natural killer cell activation in mice and men: different triggers for similar weapons?' *Nat Immunol.* 2002, Sep. 3 (9) 807–13.

- Malaviya, R., Abraham, S. N. 'Mast cell modulation of immune responses to bacteria'. *Immunol. Rev.* 2001, Feb. 179: 16–24.

- Hornef, M. W., Wick, M. J., Rhen, M., Normark, S. 'Bacterial strategies for overcoming host innate and adaptive immune responses'. *Nat. Immunol.* 2002, Nov. 3 (11) :1033–40.

- Rosenberger, C. M., Finlay, B. B. 'Phagocyte sabotage: disruption of macrophage signaling by bacterial pathogens', *Nat. Rev. Mol. Cell. Biol.* 2003, May. 4 (5): 385–96.

- Goebel, W. et al. 'Bacterial replication in the host cell cytosol'. *Curr. Opin. Micro.* 2000; 3: 49.

- Gao, L.-Y. et al. 'Modulation of host cell apoptosis by intracellular bacterial pathogens'. *Trends Micro.* 2000; 8: 306.

- Torres-Vazquez, A. et al. 'Salmonella pathogenicity island 2 dependent evasion of the phagocyte NADPH oxidase'. *Science* 2000; 287: 1655.

- Orange, J. S., Fassett, M. S., Koopman, L. A., Boyson, J. E., Strominger, J. L. 'Viral evasion of natural killer cells'. *Nat. Immunol.* 2002, Nov. 3 (11): 1006–12.

- Favoreel, H. W., van der Walle, G. R., Nauwynck, H. J. and Pensaert, M. B. 'Virus complement evasion strategies'. *J. Gen. Virol.* 2002; 84: 1.

- Mocarski, E. S. Jr. 'Immunomodulation by cytomegaloviruses: manipulative strategies beyond evasion'. *Trends Microbiol.* 2002, Jul. 10 (7): 332–9.

- Sacks, D., Sher, A. 'Evasion of innate immunity by parasitic protozoa'. *Nat. Immunol.* 2002, Nov. 3 (11): 1041–7.

- Maizels, R. M., Gomez-Escobar, N., Gregory, W. F., Murray, J., Zang, X. 'Immune evasion genes from filarial nematodes. *Int. J. Parasitol.* 2001, Jul. 31 (9): 889–98.

- Cohen, J. 'The immunopathogenesis of sepsis'. *Nature*. 2002, Dec. 19–26; 420 (6917): 885–91.

Adaptive Immunity

- Manis, J. P., Tian, M. and Alt, F. W. 'Mechanism and control of class switch recombination'. *Trends in Immunology*. 2002; 23: 31.

- Bishop, G. A. and Hostager, B. S. 'B lymphocyte activation by contact mediated interactions with T lymphocytes'. *Curr. Opin. Immunol*. 2001; 13: 278.

- Diaz, M. and Casali, P. 'Somatic immunoglobulin hypermutation'. *Curr. Opin. Immunol*. 2002; 14: 235.

- Chadd, H. E. and Chamow, S. M. 'Therapeutic antibody expression technology'. *Curr. Opin. Immunol*. 2001; 12: 188.

- Reis e Sousa, C., Sher, A., Kaye, P. 'The role of dendritic cells in the induction and regulation of immunity to microbial infection'. *Curr. Opin. Immunol*. 1999, 11 (4): 392–9.

- Kelsall, B. L., Biron, C. A., Sharma, O., Kaye, P. M. 'Dendritic cells at the host-pathogen interface'. *Nat. Immunol*. 2002, Aug, 3 (8) :699–702.

- Gordon, S. 'Alternative activation of macrophages'. *Nat. Rev. Immunol*. 2003, Jan. 3 (1): 23–35.

- van der Merwe 'Formation and function of the immunological synapse'. *Curr. Opin. Immunol*. 2002; 14: 293.

- Murphy, K. M. and Reiner, S. L. 'The lineage decisions of helper T cells'. *Nat. Rev. Immunol*. 2002; 2: 933.

- Robinson, D. S., O'Garra, A. 'Further checkpoints in Th1 development'. *Immunity*. 2002, Jun. 16 (6): 755–8.

- Vincent, M. S., Gumperz, J. E., Brenner, M. B. 'Understanding the function of CD1-restricted T cells'. *Nat. Immunol*. 2003, Jun. 4 (6): 517–23.

- Palmer, E. 'Negative selection–clearing out the bad apples from the T-cell repertoire'. *Nat. Rev. Immunol*. 2003, May. 3 (5): 383–91.

- Jameson, J., Witherden, D., Havran, W. L. 'T-cell effector mechanisms: gamma delta and CD1d-restricted subsets'. *Curr. Opin. Immunol*. 2003; Jun;15(3):349–53.

- Lieberman, J. 'The ABCs of granule-mediated cytotoxicity: new weapons in the arsenal'. *Nat. Rev. Immunol*. 2003, May. 3 (5): 361–70.

- Von Andrian, U. H. 'T cell activation in six dimensions'. *Science*. 2002; 296: 1815.

- McGuirk, P., Mills, K. H. 'Pathogen-specific regulatory T cells provoke a shift in the Th1/Th2 paradigm in immunity to infectious diseases'. *Trends. Immunol*. 2002, Sep. 23 (9): 450–5.

- Sprent, J., Surh, C. D. 'T cell memory'. *Annu. Rev. Immunol.* 2002; 20: 551–79.
- Harding, C. V., Ramachandra, L., Wick, M. J. 'Interaction of bacteria with antigen presenting cells: influences on antigen presentation and antibacterial immunity'. *Curr. Opin. Immunol.* 2003, Feb. 15 (1): 112–9.
- Hornef, M. W., Wick, M. J., Rhen, M., Normark, S. 'Bacterial strategies for overcoming host innate and adaptive immune responses'. *Nat. Immunol.* 2002, Nov. 3 (11): 1033–40.
- Yewdell, J. W., Hill, A. B. 'Viral interference with antigen presentation'. *Nat. Immunol.* 2002, Nov. 3 (11): 1019–25.
- Benedict, C. A., Norris, P. S., Ware, C. F. 'To kill or be killed: viral evasion of apoptosis'. *Nat. Immunol.* 2002, Nov. 3 (11): 1013–8.
- Zambrano-Vila, S., Rosales-Borjas, Carrero, J. C. and Ortoz-Ortiz, L. 'How protozoan parasites evade the immune response'. *Trends in Parasitology.* 2002; 18: 272.
- Collins, H. L., Kaufmann, S. H. 'The many faces of host responses to tuberculosis'. *Immunology.* 2001, May. 103 (1): 1–9.
- Rowland-Jones, S. L. 'Timeline: AIDS pathogenesis: what have two decades of HIV research taught us?' *Nat. Rev. Immunol.* 2003, Apr. 3 (4): 343–8.
- Klenerman, P., Wu, Y., Phillips, R. 'HIV: current opinion in escapology'. *Curr. Opin. Microbiol.* 2002, Aug. 5 (4): 408–13.
- Young, D., Hussell, T., Dougan, G. 'Chronic bacterial infections: living with unwanted guests'. *Nat. Immunol.* 2002, Nov. 3 (11): 1026–32.
- Wills-Karp, M., Santeliz, J. and Karp, C. L. 'The germless theory of allergic disease: revisiting the hygiene hypothesis'. *Nat. Rev. Immunol.* 2001; 1: 69.
- Chapel, H., Geha, R., Rosen, F. 'Primary immunodeficiency diseases: an update'. IUIS PID (Primary Immunodeficiencies) Classification committee. *Clin. Exp. Immunol.* 2003, Apr. 132 (1): 9–15.
- Hacein-Bey-Abina, S., von Kalle, C., Schmidt, M., Le Deist Wulffraat, N., McIntyre, E., Radford, I., Villeval, J. L., Fraser, C. C., Cavazzana-Calvo, M., Fischer, A. 'A serious adverse event after successful gene therapy for X-linked severe combined immunodeficiency'. *N. Engl. J. Med.* 2003, Jan. 16: 348 (3): 255–6.

Part 3   The host-pathogen balance

Textbooks

- Giesecke, J. *Modern Infectious Disease Epidemiology.* Edward Arnold, 2nd edn. 2002.

- Plotkin S. A., Orenstein W. A. (eds.) *Vaccines*. Saunders 4th edn 2004.
- Scholar, E. M. and Pratt, W. B. *The Antimicrobial drugs*. 2nd edn. Oxford University Press. 2000.
- Bell D. *Lecture notes on Tropical Medicine*. Oxford, Blackwell. 5th edn. (2003).
- *Hunter's Tropical Medicine*. Philadelphia, W. B. Saunders, 8th edn. (2000).

Websites:

- www.bmn.com/infectious-diseases (BioMedNet gateway to reviews and articles in infectious diseases.)
- www.who.int/health_topics/hiv_infections/en/ (WHO HIV Infections web site:)
- www.unaids.org/ (The Joint United Nations Programme on HIV/AIDS.)
- www.who.int/health-topics/tb.htm (WHO Tuberculosis web site)
- www.cdc.gov/ncidod/diseases/eid/index.htm (CDC Emerging Infectious Diseases Web site:)
- www.cdc.gov/nip/publications/pink (Epidemiology and prevention of vaccine-preventable diseases.)
- www.cdc.gov/nip (has general information on vaccine schedules.)
- www.who.int.ith (a good chapter on vaccine preventable diseases.)
- www.vaccinealliance.org/home/index.php (the Global Alliance for Vaccines and Immunization (GAVI) website.)

Recent Reviews and Articles:

- Collins, H. L., Kaufmann, S. H. 'Prospects for better tuberculosis vaccines'. *Lancet Infect. Dis.* 2001, Aug. 1 (1): 21–8.
- Williamson, E. D., Titball, R. W. 'Vaccines against dangerous pathogens'. *Br. Med. Bull.* 2002; 62: 163–73.
- Moorthy, V., Hill, A. V. 'Malaria vaccines'. *Br. Med. Bull.* 2002; 62: 59–72.
- Mwau, M., McMichael, A. J. 'A review of vaccines for HIV prevention'. *J. Gene Med.* 2003, Jan.–Feb. 5 (1): 3–10.
- Martin, B., Nelson, M., Hershey, J., Engler, R. 'Adverse reactions to vaccines'. *Clin. Rev. Allergy Immunol.* 2003, Jun. 24 (3): 263–76.
- Cooke, G. S., Hill, A. V. 'Genetics of susceptibility to human infectious disease'. *Nat. Rev. Genet.* 2001, Dec. 2 (12): 967–77.
- Livermore, D. M. 'Bacterial resistance: origins, epidemiology, and impact'. *Clin. Infect. Dis.* 2003, Jan. 15; 36 (Suppl 1): S11–23.
- Beeching, N. J., Dance, D. A., Miller, A. R., Spencer, R. C. 'Biological warfare and bioterrorism'. *BMJ.* 2002, Feb. 9; 324 (7333): 336–9.

Index

Numbers in **bold face** refer to figures or tables